High

High

Six Principles
for Guilt-Free Pleasure
and Escape

Jodie Gould

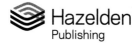

Hazelden
Publishing

Hazelden Publishing
Center City, Minnesota 55012
hazelden.org/bookstore

Cover design: Theresa Jaeger Gedig
Page design: Ann Delgehausen, Trio Bookworks

About Hazelden Publishing

As part of the Hazelden Betty Ford Foundation, Hazelden Publishing offers both cutting-edge educational resources and inspirational books. Our print and digital works help guide individuals in treatment and recovery, and their loved ones. Professionals who work to prevent and treat addiction also turn to Hazelden Publishing for evidence-based curricula, digital content solutions, and videos for use in schools, treatment programs, correctional programs, and electronic health records systems. We also offer training for implementation of our curricula. Through published and digital works, Hazelden Publishing extends the reach of healing and hope to individuals, families, and communities affected by addiction and related issues.

For more information about Hazelden publications, please call **800-328-9000** or visit us online at **hazelden.org/bookstore**.

To my daughter, Samantha,
who makes me feel high every single day!

Contents

Part Two

The Six Pleasure Principles

Acknowledgments

To Linda Konner, for being the best agent and friend a person can have. To my editor, Sid Farrar, for coming up with the concept of this book and for allowing me to run with it, and for his keen editorial skills and guidance. And to everyone on the Hazelden team (marketing, publicity, sales, production, and support staff): I was you in a past life; I know how hard you work to get books like this one into the right hands.

of snowy white powder within reach. Williams had recently gone to a treatment facility for a "recharge" and appeared to be sober and stable when his body, with a belt around his neck, was found by his personal assistant. Sadly, Hoffman and Williams are just two of the far too many gifted artists whose lives have been devastated by alcohol and other drugs—not to mention the tens of thousands of regular folks who succumb to the siren call of addiction every year. But this book is not about people like Hoffman and Williams—addicts who use in spite of the dangers to their health and the collateral damage to family and friends. *High* is primarily for and about people who might have experimented with drugs in the past (like me) and people who are doing so now (perhaps you or someone you know). It is for those, like me, who enjoy a glass or two of wine with dinner or with friends; those who might like a puff of pot to relax or to flex their creative muscles; and those who pop the occasional prescription anti-anxiety pill to help take the edge off an uncomfortable situation—none of which necessarily makes them candidates for intervention.

This book is about the healthier choices that we can make to achieve the same results we're usually seeking when we turn to drugs and alcohol in the first place: to relax, have fun, relieve pain, and de-stress. Yes, I drink wine with dinner, but I also practice yoga regularly; meditate (okay, not as often as I should, but I try); spin (indoor cycle) three days a week; take breaks from endless hours staring at this blasted computer screen to walk in the park or around my neighborhood; dance with abandon with my teenage daughter to some ear-wormy pop music in the privacy of our living room so not to mortify her; regularly stay in touch with or visit my family; and make lunch or dinner dates with friends. Although my clubbing days are over—and yes, they were fun—I can honestly say that as a middle-aged mom, I am far healthier than I was when I was a cigarette-smoking, bar-hopping youth. While my cares have increased through the years (financial concerns, failing health of friends and family members, worries about the safety, education and well-being of my child), I've found better ways to cope with life's inevitable pain and anxiety.

It is important to acknowledge that our never-ending quest for pleasure and escape is an indelible part of our nature. Our walks on the wild side do not have to cause us shame or self-loathing. In fact, as you will learn, this natural craving is something that we share with our fellow creatures, including cats, dogs, birds, horses, elephants, and dolphins. But what we also share with many animals is the pleasure we get from food, family, play, and companionship. Elephants, for example, live in tight-knit units. They have been observed exhibiting emotions like joy, compassion, and grief, and they even appear to get pleasure from listening to music and from painting.

You will see how the need to pursue an altered state of consciousness is also deeply rooted in human history, dating back millions of years, from prehistoric times when cave dwellers first discovered fermented drinks, to the meth labs and painkiller pill mills of today. By taking a look at our biological, psychological, and historical desire to get high, we might better understand that these desires are yet another drive, much like hunger, thirst, or sex.

Clearly, our getting high is not necessary for our survival and, in the case of addiction, can actually threaten it, but it is a natural urge nonetheless. And like other drives, the desire for intoxication has no social or economic boundaries, coursing as liberally through slums and trailer parks as through suburbs and gated communities, as well as the halls of government, business, and higher education. In fact, some our greatest minds, including philosophers, writers, artists, and innovators, have been active users of drugs and alcohol. They include Sigmund Freud, who was a compulsive cigar smoker and had a taste for cocaine; the poet John Keats, whose musings were said to be influenced by opium; and Michel Foucault, the French social theorist who wrote about a spectacular acid trip in Death Valley, California, which he described as "the greatest experience of his life."

All this begs a question that is an underlying theme of this book: What is behind this universal need to engage in mind-altering pleasure? One explanation is really quite simple—getting high usually makes us feel better than we do when we aren't. Whether it's purely recreational or whether it's an attempt to relieve physical pain, depression, or hardship, the use of alcohol and other drugs has been and always will be a go-to option. But what else can we do to escape the boredom and inevitable pain and sadness that we all sometimes feel during our lives? How can we find pleasure or simply experience the joy in living?

Because tragedies like Hoffman's and Williams's will continue to occur, it is important to keep in mind that besides the drugs smuggled, injected, snorted, or bought from the neighborhood dealer that make dramatic news stories, there are mood-altering substances so pervasive in our lives that many of us are not even aware of how dependent we are on them. Do you crave that cup of coffee when you wake up in the morning? Do you take hourly cigarette breaks? Do you knock back pints of beer or take a few tokes of pot with your buddies after work? Do you relax with a cocktail after the kids are safely tucked away in bed, or are you a fan of momtini play dates, where alcoholic beverages are as ubiquitous as juice boxes? Can you go to a social function without popping a Valium first? Are you able to drift off to sleep without an Ambien?

However it is you choose to alter your mood, I invite you to explore what getting high is all about and learn how you can fulfill this natural desire to transcend everyday life in ways that expand your consciousness naturally, without harming your mind, body, and spirit. Read on, and you will discover:

- The history of the human pursuit of an altered state of consciousness—from the Stone Age and the Age of Aquarius to today's club drugs and 4:20 festivals, and how our attitudes toward drugs and pleasure-seeking have evolved over the years. Whether legal or not, the substances we use change with the times—new ones are added, old ones make comebacks, and some, like alcohol, have been around just about forever. Whatever the drug or drink du jour, history tells us our quest for pleasure and escape will never cease.

- The part our brain plays in our desire to relieve pain and depression, how its function as a sophisticated processor of chemicals is part our drive to self-medicate, and ways that we can change our brain to give us pleasure.

- What some animals do to get high and how they also find similar pleasure and comfort in the natural activities of eating, playing, bonding, and nurturing.

- How philosophers have defined pleasure and its pursuit.

- The six Pleasure Principles, which are:
  1. *Move* (inhabiting the body through physical activity);
  2. *Restore* (revitalizing mind, body, and spirit);

3. *Connect* (bonding with family, friends, and community);

4. *Create* (expressing and expanding the inner self);

5. *Celebrate* (affirming life, experiencing joy); and

6. *Give* (being of service, finding purpose).

These Pleasure Principles, which include proven methods for reducing depression and anxiety and enhancing well-being, will help you find that the best highs come from being fully present and alive. Studies have shown a correlation between these principles and longevity, so not only will you feel better by engaging in these life-affirming behaviors—not to mention avoiding the hangovers and other side effects of drugs—you might even live longer.

Part One

Getting High

1

Doing It Old School
The History of Getting High

The harvesting and selling of mood-altering substances may not be the world's oldest profession, but using them is undoubtedly one of the oldest forms of recreation. Anthropologists say it didn't take long for Paleolithic people to discover how to turn plants into inebriating beverages and potions—which probably made a life of hunting and gathering more tolerable on the one hand and created more tribal fighting on the other. And as you'll see in chapter 3, our forebears learned how to get high by imitating the primates and other animals that feasted on fermented fruits and hallucinogenic plants.

From the Babylonians to Prohibition

The earliest evidence of prehistoric tippling can be seen on cave paintings (a form of creative expression, one of the healthier pleasures that I will discuss in part 2) that depict the collection of honey, which was fermented and made into an intoxicating beverage. Beer eventually became popular with the Babylonians around 2700 BCE and was offered to goddesses and other deities, since the Babylonians believed the gods also liked to party. Recipes for beer have been found on clay tablets, and Mesopotamian art also depicts our ancestors drinking beer from large vats and pots.

All across the ancient world people were getting high from fermented drinks traded throughout Greece, Rome, Egypt, Mesopotamia, and Iron Age Europe. The Egyptians, whose contributions to civilization are legendary, developed a technique for brewing beer from barley and emmer wheat before they learned how to make bread. (Apparently, early humans could live on beer alone.) They worshiped Osiris, the god of beer, and they brewed beer at home, sometimes on a daily basis.

RAISING CANE (SUGAR)

A scientific side note: The sugar fermentation process, called glycolysis, produces alcohol when yeast interacts with sugar, which is the result of the natural metabolic breakdown of rotting fruit. Early humans used their environment as nature's distillery, turning grains into beer, wine, and spirits. Many of the wild fruits and foods collected by hunter-gatherers had high sugar content and could be fermented into an intoxicating drink. Although beer is older, wine became the most popular alcoholic beverage during the Neolithic period and was stored in ceramic containers, jars, stone bowls, and sometimes the cavities in rocks.

Biblical Boozing

Although today drinking is prohibited by certain religions such as Mormonism, Seventh Day Adventism, Buddhism, and Islam, some ancient people saw spirits as a holy conduit in their offerings to the gods. While altered states of consciousness could be achieved by fasting or meditation, alcohol was used by shamans to escape the mundane, as many people do today, and to tackle the larger questions about the meaning of life.

The Bible is rife with tales of drinking, including one passage that recommends giving alcohol to those who are dying or depressed so they can forget their misery: "Let beer be for those who are perishing, wine for those who are in anguish! Let them drink and forget their poverty and remember their misery no more" (Proverbs 31:6–7, New International Version).

However compassionate offering libations to the suffering might be, the Bible is not as lenient when it comes to drunkenness, warning that intoxication can lead to lapses in morality, sexual misconduct, and sloth: "Do not join those who drink too much wine or gorge themselves on meat, for drunkards and gluttons become poor, and drowsiness clothes them in rags" (Proverbs 23:20–21, NIV).

One of the most well-known biblical boozers was Noah, whose unwavering faith while living in a society drenched in chaos and rebellion was said to have pleased God. According to Genesis, Noah had a weakness for wine. After the floodwaters receded and his animal passengers repopulated the land, Noah was said to have observed a goat frolicking while eating fermented grapes. He decided to give it a try. The multicentenarian (in biblical years) became tipsy and broke into jubilant song.

It seems Noah was a blackout drunk, because the Old Testament describes how he shed his clothes during his revelry and ended up crashing naked: "When he drank some of its wine, he became drunk and lay uncovered inside his tent" (Genesis 9:21, NIV). The next morning, he confessed to his sons about what happened, and despite his shame about his only sin, the booze-besotted Noah replanted the grapevine in his garden.

The Bible isn't the only holy book to extol the virtues of spirits and to caution against their pitfalls. According to some Hindu texts, alcohol is said to improve one's digestion, respiratory system, voice, and intelligence. Despite this belief in the health benefits of moderate alcohol use, J. V. Hebbar, a modern-day physician specializing in Ayurvedic medicine, warns people with anger or fear issues, excessive thirst or hunger, or severe grief or panic attacks, and those who are tired from traveling or too much exercise, to avoid liquor.

Archeologists Dig It

As civilizations grew, people continued to celebrate and self-medicate with alcohol and other drugs. One recent excavation in Israel uncovered the ruins of the largest wine cellar ever found, buried beneath a Canaanite palace circa 1700 BCE. The cellar contained the equivalent of 3,000 bottles of red and white wines, which is a lot of historic hooch. Both the Greeks and the Romans generally drank diluted wine at breakfast and formal symposiums.

Another archeological dig found even older jugs used for fermented beer from around 10,000 BCE. Chemical analysis of the microscopic residue on the containers led researchers to identify the contents of archaic brews.

While ancient people clearly loved their libations, plants containing psychoactive ingredients were also chewed, smoked, swallowed, and sniffed. Opium, for example, made from poppies, was used in Mesopotamia five thousand years ago—its medicinal properties chronicled on cuneiform tablets. The Greek poet Homer described in his epic *The Odyssey* the brewing and offering of an opium tea as a beverage of hospitality, which caused warriors to have strange and terrifying hallucinations. Real-life Greek soldiers used opium before going into battle; sacking and pillaging was a rough and risky endeavor.

Modern-day proponents of medical marijuana might not be surprised to learn that ancient Chinese practitioners prescribed cannabis for a variety of conditions, including gout, rheumatism, malaria, loss of appetite, and constipation, and as an aid in childbirth. The ancient Hindu sages of India also considered marijuana an indispensable part of religious life.

Veni Vidi Vino

After important dinners and symposiums (some of which presumably involved sumptuous banquets with castratos fanning guests with palm fronds), Romans would sometimes indulge in a game of *convivium*, which sounds a lot more congenial than it actually was. The rules were simple but strict. To start, the host determined how much everyone was going to drink (anywhere from one to eleven glasses of alcohol). Next, like a game of boozy Russian roulette, everyone took turns drinking. And while staying in the contest reaped few rewards (other than a reputation for being able to hold your liquor), being voted out had social repercussions. If you couldn't keep up or keep down your liquor, if you passed or passed out, or even burped during the rounds, you would be banned from joining a future *convivium*. And since only the crème de la crème were invited, getting banished was the equivalent to getting banished from the cool kids' table.

Ouzo Boozo

It is an ancient Greek tradition to break a glass after making a toast (not encouraged in modern restaurants, of course). A glass might well have been filled with ouzo: a combination of pressed grapes, herbs, and berries that is still enjoyed today. The idea was to prevent the glass from being used for a lesser tribute. This ritual is usually followed by a rousing *"opa!"* or possibly a circle dance of celebrants. (See the film *Zorba the Greek* for a visual reference.) Way back in the day, there was also a game called *kottabos*, where, like an ancient version of beer pong, participants would toss the dregs of their drinks at a target in the middle of the room. They were judged on whether they hit the target—a disk balanced on a narrow stand (like a pole)— and also on their throwing form. By hitting the mark they could win prizes such as baked goods and kisses from servers. According to one source, many Greeks took as much pride in playing *kottabos* as others did in hurling the javelin, although my guess is that there was another type of hurling going on by the time this game was over.

Medieval Medication

The Middle Ages was not known as a carefree, fun-loving period, but medieval people did shed their armor from time to time, especially in Europe, where cider and pomace wine were enjoyed by peasant and landowner alike. Even nuns, bless their hearts, were allowed six pints of ale each day. Wine made from grapes, however, was preferred by the upper classes (swirl and sniff). Around 1250, Europeans developed the process of distillation and added brandy and other liquors to the spirits list. The generic term for these distilled products was *aqua vitae,* or "the water of life."

While actual water remained the most popular drink during the Middle Ages, chiefly because it was free and accessible (Evian had not yet been invented), beer provided much-needed calories for laborers and farmers. (Ale was to laborers what Gatorade is to pro athletes.) Wine was also produced all over Europe, but it was expensive and beyond the means of most ordinary people. Tavern owners would buy it in bulk and sell it to the pedestrian patrons by the cup. While inns provided lodging for wealthier travelers, taverns were for drinking and myriad amusements such as gambling, singing, and procuring prostitutes.

People would also gather at a neighbor's house for batches of ale. Inevitably, fights and fatal accidents often followed a session of drinking. According to one twelfth-century court record, the son of William Cristmasse returned home around midnight "drunk and disgustingly over-fed," where he died after tripping and breaking his skull. Another man perished after falling off his horse while galloping home from the tavern—a victim of drunk riding. And yet another unfortunate fellow was reported to have urinated in a pond before falling in and drowning. (Talk about pissing life away.)

Dark Ages Jug Heads

During the 1300s across the English Channel in France, a Gallic drinking game was designed to test the agility of patrons. It was also an amusing way to make drunks look like idiots. The game worked like this: so-called puzzle jugs (jugs with holes punched in them) were partially filled with wine; if a tippler didn't tilt the jug in precisely the right way while covering up the holes with his fingers, the contents would spill out. In addition to this being a knee-slapper, barflies often gambled on whether a new rube had the chops to get the wine from jug to mouth without spilling. More often than not, the contents ended up in the player's lap. This humiliating game remained a popular barroom feature for the next four hundred years.

Elizabethan Inebriation

Elizabethans were a deeply class-conscious society, where drinking to excess was either tolerated or abhorred depending on one's status. Drunkenness among the wealthy was considered a private vice, while intoxication among the commoners was said to increase crime, undermine gender roles, and destroy family values.

This paradox created a dilemma for writer and social conservative Henry Fielding, author of the satirical novel *Tom Jones*, whose views reflected this separation between those of the manor born and impoverished "drunkards." Fielding's belief that "the upper part of life" should be distinguished from the lower meant that immorality among the rich should remain beyond the reach of the legal system, while the same behavior among the poor presented a serious threat to civilized society.

Of course, Britons of lesser means drank to escape the drudgery of daily life, especially Londoners who lived in crowded, putrid conditions surrounded by the stench of refuse. (Chamber pots were emptied out of windows, and there was no drainage system, for example.) Tea had not yet become popular, and people drank water only if they couldn't afford to buy ale. César de Saussure, a Swiss visitor to England in the 1720s, observed, "Though water is to be had in abundance in London . . . absolutely none is drunk. In this country beer is what everybody drinks when thirsty."

Back in seventeenth-century England, drinking was sometimes followed by swearing one's allegiance to king and country. Rollicking royalists would try to one-up their drinking buddies by literally putting their asses on the line. After they sang drunken ballads to His Highness and the church, the ribaldry would devolve into what amounted to a game of truth or derriere, where the most loyal among them would slice off a piece of their butt and then toast their own blood to the monarchy. As you can imagine, this game would frequently go horribly wrong, given that drunks wielding knives is never a good idea.

The Puritans

Contrary to popular belief, Protestant leaders such as Martin Luther and John Calvin believed alcohol was a gift from God that was to be used in moderation for pleasure, enjoyment, and health. Drunkenness was viewed as a sin but was nevertheless a part of everyday life. This explains why the cargo in the Mayflower contained more beer than water. In addition to avoiding safety issues with water contamination, alcohol also enhanced one's attitude toward life, which was tough going for even the hardiest of pilgrims.

Of course, the English had been drinking beer for centuries, so colonial men and women were more than happy to carry on the tradition and drank it often, including with meals. Because importing beer was costly, the early settlers started brewing their own. The results were bitter, given the inhospitable harvesting conditions. Eventually, seeds were imported from England in order to cultivate a supply of better-tasting beer.

But the longer people remained in the colonies, the further they drifted from their beer-drinking heritage. By the end of the seventeenth century, Americans switched to rum, which originated in Barbados. According to a visiting English writer, Edward Ward, rum was "adored" by the American English: "'Tis held as the comforter of their souls, the preserver of their bodies, the remover of their cares, and promoter of their mirth; and is a sovereign remedy against the grumbling of the guts."

Tobacco: America's Cash Crop

One cannot chronicle the history of drugs without mentioning tobacco, which the first English settlers puffed in Virginia, thanks to pipe-smoking Native Americans. Over the next 160 years, tobacco would become one of America's biggest cash crops. Later generations became hooked on the cigarette's most addictive ingredient: nicotine. The cancer-causing effects of tar and nicotine were not fully realized until medical studies were done in the mid-twentieth century and were eventually revealed despite a cover-up by tobacco companies.

In the mid-nineteenth century, two prominent physicians championed smoking as a treatment for asthma. One of these geniuses, Henry Hyde Salter, believed that asthma was caused by nervousness or excitement, which led to spasms of the bronchial tube muscles. He advocated a range of so-called treatments, including smoking tobacco and taking sedatives such as chloroform and stramonium to relieve and suppress irritation. One wonders how long the patients of these doctors survived.

A recent study conducted by far smarter researchers at Columbia University and the Centre for Addiction and Mental Health in Toronto found that nicotine also makes people more susceptible to drug addiction. Surveys found that 97 percent of cocaine users smoked cigarettes before trying coke, making nicotine a primary gateway drug.

Prohibition

By the 1820s Americans drank seven gallons of alcohol per person annually—in part because whiskey was cheap to produce. The growing rates of crime, poverty, and infant mortality during the industrial revolution were often attributed to the scourge of alcohol. The seemingly gaping maw of overindulgence gave birth to the temperance movement, spearheaded chiefly by women and religious leaders who proselytized by enumerating the evils of booze. The movement eventually ushered in Prohibition in 1920, when the Eighteenth Amendment to the Constitution was adopted, banning the manufacture, transportation, and sale of liquor. Surprisingly, the enforcement of Prohibition was originally assigned to the IRS—just one of many reasons the Eighteenth Amendment was doomed to failure. Not so shocking is that Prohibition was nearly impossible to enforce, and almost overnight, America became the land of criminal opportunity. Alcohol sales and use were driven underground, creating a well-spring of gangland violence, bootleggers, and illegal drinking clubs. While the actual number of speakeasies is not known, the New York Historical Society estimates it ranged from twenty thousand to a hundred thousand in New York City alone. Prohibition was repealed with the passage of the Twenty-First Amendment on December 5, 1933, to many Americans' relief.

THE WRATH OF GRAPES

Born in 1846, the uniquely named Carry Nation earned a reputation (admired by some, detested by others) as an anti-alcohol vigilante. A formidable six feet tall and clad in modest black-and-white garb, Nation would bar-storm across Kansas and Oklahoma, often accompanied by a hymn-singing, hatchet-swinging posse, with whom she would smash every glass, light fixture, and bottle in sight. She even appeared in the Kansas governor's chambers to rail against the evils of liquor.

Alcohol was not her only enemy. Nation despised tobacco, foreign cuisine (what do those foreigners know about good cookin'?), corsets (well, she might have had a point there), short skirts (one assumes dresses that exposed an ankle), and fraternal orders (i.e., men's clubs—she might have had a point with that one as well). Her anti-booze and anti-tobacco fervor was rumored to have stemmed from a short-lived marriage to an alcoholic. Less than a decade after her death, the temperance movement that was her cause célèbre finally succeeded, and the hard-drinking country had gone officially dry.

The Pharma Revolution

When you think of drug lords, images of ruthless capos (or Walt in HBO's *Breaking Bad*) might come to mind. But history shows that drug kingpins might also wear pinstriped suits. The fact is, many illegal drugs today were first marketed by pharmaceutical companies, and legal drug sales in the United States now far exceed what's made on the black market. In the nineteenth and early twentieth centuries, people suffering from any number of diseases and bodily discomforts could find what was touted as cures at their local pharmacy. Heroin, for example, was invented by Bayer Pharmaceuticals in 1898 and sold for use in cough syrup during an age of rampant pneumonia and tuberculosis. Around 1899, stories about addiction cases started to spread as fast as these diseases. Subsequently, Bayer ceased production of heroin in 1913, and it was banned in the United States in 1924.

Cocaine and methamphetamine were also offered as elixirs for everything from sore throats and toothaches to coughs, insomnia, and depression. And though the idea of giving children cocaine to relieve a toothache would now result in a call to Child Protection Services, the drug's use as an over-the-counter medication was acceptable from the 1880s until the beginning of the twentieth century. Sigmund Freud extolled the virtues of cocaine as a treatment for depression and impotence.

During this period, beverages and tonics also contained cocaine. Coca-Cola's initial popularity (along with its name) may well have been due to the drug's inclusion among the soda's ingredients. Long-term users may have suffered from disrupted eating and sleeping patterns, psychotic delusions, hallucinations, and severe depression upon withdrawal. Cocaine was banned in the United States in 1920, but by then the drug had already been coursing through the veins of the general public for years.

In 1849, the demure-sounding Mrs. Charlotte N. Winslow of Maine launched her Soothing Syrup, a chemical cocktail of sodium carbonate, aqua ammonia, and sixty-five milligrams of morphine per fluid ounce. The syrup was advertised as a medicine for tots who were teething, and one mother wrote to the *New York Times* lauding its "magical" effect on her son. "He soon went to sleep," she says, "and all pain and nervousness disappeared." No kidding. The American Medical Association had a different take on this syrup, denouncing it as a "baby killer" in 1911, although it remained on the market until 1930.

Another powerful narcotic called laudanum, an alcoholic mixture containing 10 percent powdered opium, was used in the 1800s to treat everything from meningitis and menstrual cramps to yellow fever. Once again, babies were spoon-fed the drug, which the manufacturer of Atkinson and Barker's Royal Infants' Preservative claimed in advertisements to relieve teething pain, bowel problems, flatulence, and convulsions. What it failed to mention was that, aside from its addictive properties, laudanum can also cause constipation, itching, and respiratory distress. Although it is still available, the drug's use is restricted.

Along with these toxic substances was a drug called Norodin, one of the most frightening medicines to be legally sold as a brand name for methamphetamine. The producers of Norodin claimed it was "useful in dispelling the shadows of mild mental depression" and that it had "relatively few side effects," if you don't count the rotting teeth, paranoia, flesh crawling sensation, and potential brain damage.

Getting High in the Modern Era

During the thirties, the propaganda against marijuana included the cautionary-turned-cult-film *Reefer Madness* that showed potheads going rogue and, eventually, criminally insane. Still, artists, poets, writers, and musicians continued to smoke weed, which they felt increased their sensitivity and creativity. Songs like "When I Get Low, I Get High" (Ella Fitzgerald), "Viper's Drag" (Fats Waller), and "Reefer Man" (Cab Calloway) were all anthems to pot and other mood-altering substances.

After World War II, the pharmaceutical industry introduced a slew of new drugs to prevent and cure disease, alleviate pain, keep you awake, help you sleep, and reduce anxiety. Thanks to Madison Avenue's media campaigns, including DuPont's "Better living through chemistry," medicine cabinets across America were filled with prescriptions for every kind of ailment.

During the fifties, heroin was increasingly seen as a hard drug used by junkies, although many middle-class kids tried it, and some got hooked. But the Beats (short for "Beatniks"), who lived in New York's Greenwich Village and other counterculture meccas, were smoking and singing about weed, sometimes in thinly veiled terms (e.g., Bob Dylan's "Rainy Day Woman," the chorus of which states, "Everybody must get stoned").

By the 1960s many illegal drugs were seen by young people in rebellion against the Vietnam War and mainstream values not as evil or dangerous but as a way to expand one's mind and reject the definition of success (i.e., get a good job, get married, have 2.5 kids) that their parents and grandparents espoused. Pot, acid, mushrooms, hash, and quaaludes were all an accepted part of a growing youth culture. Soldiers barely out of their teens were being drafted to fight in an intensely unpopular war, and many of them used everything they could get their hands on to help ease their pain and horror.

Timothy Leary, who earned his doctorate in psychology at the University of California, Berkeley, launched the Harvard Psilocybin Project in 1965. The goal of Leary's research was to analyze the effects of a synthesized version of psilocybin mushrooms on humans, in hopes of discovering better methods for treating alcoholism and to reform convicted criminals. He decided to experiment by taking the drug himself, which eventually led Leary to promote LSD for personal enlightenment. Speaking at the San Francisco "Be-In" in 1967, he delivered the phrase that became the credo of the decade: "Turn on, tune in, drop out." As acid became widely available on the black market, many users were hospitalized following bad trips that resulted from overdoses or contamination. Some reported having acid flashbacks weeks or even months after tripping. The use of LSD plummeted by the mid-eighties.

Luke, Age Sixty-Four, Copywriter from Connecticut

I was drafted to Vietnam when I was twenty-one.
The war was extremely unpopular in the States, so the morale when I got there was absolutely horrible. A lot of us were draftees. One day we were walking down the street, and a month later we're in the jungle. All we wanted to do was get it done and go home.

Drugs and alcohol were everywhere, and I did a little bit of everything, but mostly I smoked weed.

A lot of soldiers got drunk and smoked pot. LSD and psilocybin were sent in from the states. Opium you could get from Thailand. There was also a lot of high-grade heroin, which was so strong that you could smoke it at the end of a cigarette and get addicted. Heroin made you feel mellow, calm, and good. It is so insidious and powerful. I've gone through a lot of pain since 'Nam, but I avoid anything that is an opiate. I respect them, but they scare me. We would get heroin from medics, the locals, and the black market.

The terrible part was seeing these young guys turn into junkies within a matter of months. I was in one unit with a twenty-two-year-old guy who got strung out on heroin. He was the nicest guy, but you couldn't talk him out of it—you couldn't even talk to him. When I last saw him, he was really desperate. We tried to get him into a program. I don't know if he ever did get into rehab because I was transferred to another unit.

Drugs took me out of the war for a while. It was also a way to rebel against the army for putting me in this situation. A lot of guys did barbiturates. The pills were a really bad idea because they'd put you out of commission. On the other side of the coin, there was a liquid amphetamine, which was a cough syrup made for weight loss. I never tried that because it looked disgusting. There were enlisted men's clubs on the bases where guys would go to get completely hammered. In 'Nam they had hard liquor, but at the enlisted men's clubs you would have to mix it with cola. If you got hit by the enemy, you would hope that the guys were smoking weed, because they could straighten up immediately and do their jobs. The guys who were drunk or strung out on heroin would just stumble around.

When we first got back from 'Nam, nobody wanted
to know us except our friends and family. Jobs were
scarce, and people were turning their backs on us. A lot
of the guys got addicted because they were wounded
in battle and needed drugs to treat their injuries. I
knew guys who went into bars to pick up girls, who
would ask, "How many babies did you kill?" Now I get,
"Thank you for your service." So the vets would hang
out together, drink some beers, smoke a joint, and
tell war stories. I stopped using all drugs on my own.
I saw people taking downers and crashing their cars. I
thought it was idiotic.

Sex, Drugs, and Rock 'n' Roll

When the Vietnam War ended, disco briefly eclipsed rock
and roll on the radio, and later hip-hop emerged as a musical art form. Clubs like Studio 54, a New York hot spot for
the rich and famous, had lines of wannabes snaking outside its heavily guarded doors. Inside, equally long lines
of cocaine were snorted by many patrons. Plato's Retreat,
another popular Manhattan club, had a back room filled
with mattresses not intended for sleeping. Swinging, "key
parties," or mate swapping was all the rage among a certain
crowd, as were those fashion Chernobyls, the polyester shirt
and white suit, as seen in *Saturday Night Fever*. Discerning
druggies wore their coke spoons around their necks or car-
ried the powder in silver cases.

Hip-hop started in the Bronx—more precisely, according to the *New York Times*, at 1520 Sedgwick Avenue, where
DJ Kool Herc presided over the record-scratching, music-
making parties held in the basement community room.
Eventually, the spoken-word phenom spread to the suburbs, with white kids adopting (or attempting to mimic)

hip-hop's style, slang, and swagger. Lyrics often glorified drug use and, in some cases, gang wars, which brought down many a rap legend. Hip-hop culture has since cleaned up and toned down its street cred; Snoop Lion and Jay-Z are two current examples of transformed hip-hop royalty.

Other drugs that have gone the way of the disco ball include PCP, or "angel dust," a veterinary drug used recreationally. It was called "the most dangerous new drug" by *People* magazine in 1978. Darvocet was the pain pill of choice until the FDA (Food and Drug Administration) asked that it be pulled from shelves, and Tuinal, another barbiturate, stayed in vogue up until its manufacturer, Eli Lilly and Company, suspended production. Like its sister drug Tuinal, Seconal was prescribed to treat insomnia. It was also known as "dolls," after which Jacqueline Susann named her famous valley girl novel, and it sent Judy Garland and Beatles manager Brian Epstein, among others, into a permanent slumber.

Quaaludes made a revival, reaching their zenith in the seventies with an estimated four million prescriptions written each year. Congress eventually crushed the disco biscuit after categorizing quaaludes as one of the twenty most dangerous drugs.

Leah, Age Fifty-Six,
Yoga Instructor from New Jersey

I did a lot of drugs during the seventies, but my friends and I were downer freaks. We'd take lots of quaaludes and Tuinals. I loved getting high on those. If we were lucky, we'd score Seconal. To get drugs you would have to go to seedier parts of Brooklyn, where I grew up, and the dealers were all on heroin or methadone. They would sell bootleg pills that gave you all kinds of side effects like shaking. Somebody told me they put rat poison in it, but we would do anything to get high back then. We were bored teenagers.

Like the stock market, drugs in the eighties seemed to tick up, with amphetamines reversing the ever popular downer trend. Used in World War II to keep soldiers alert during battle, amphetamines made a comeback particularly with professional athletes and truck drivers. In 1982 Ronald Reagan signed an executive order mandating drug tests for truck drivers, and by 2006 Major League Baseball banned them, but performance-enhancing drugs became all the rage nevertheless.

Crack entered the illegal market around 1984. Most crackheads smoked the rock-like substance in pipes. Like the Lay's potato chips of drugs, crack is difficult to toke just once. And being a street drug used mostly by poor people of color versus a Wall Street drug used mostly by whites in suits, the penalties for selling and using were a lot stricter than those for its powdery cousin. Crack has some nasty side effects, including lung damage, respiratory problems, and increased blood pressure.

Another group of popular drugs during the high-flying eighties was amyl nitrates, or "poppers," which were known to enhance sexual pleasure by causing, among other things, the sphincter and vaginal muscles to relax. A 1978 *Time* article traced the increased use of poppers to gay men; the drug was also picked up by experimenting heteros. By 1987, 3 percent of the American population was inhaling poppers. Though popper use continued briefly into the '90s as part of the rave scene, a government crackdown was the final buzzkill. Suddenly the tiny amber bottles became impossible to score. Rumors about the connection between amyl nitrates and AIDS also put the kibosh on the popper craze.

Deirdre, Age Fifty-Five, Publicist from New York

I grew up in a volatile house where my father was an alcoholic and abusive both physically and mentally. My life was miserable, which is why I took barbiturates when I was in middle school—I needed something that would calm me down. I got them from my older brother. In high school I started going out with a guy who smoked weed. I didn't smoke anything—not even cigarettes. I hated the smell. It stayed that way until the mid-80s, when cocaine came along. With pills I knew when to stop. With coke I just wanted more.

We got into it from a retired cop who would give us bricks to sell. I would be the one to give "tastes" to the customers. I had to sleep with a bottle of Afrin under the pillow because I couldn't breathe at night. I eventually lost all the cartilage in my nose. We would play these all-night Trivial Pursuit games with another couple who were cokeheads and big Wall Street executives. We had a standing date every Friday from around five p.m. until six a.m. They would buy an ounce of coke each week. He'd go to work with an ammunition belt with little vials of coke in each bullet casing! My boyfriend and I would go back home at dawn and sleep all day. We couldn't have sex, even though we tried, because we were too strung out. It was crazy. It got to the point where I would dread Friday nights.

With the economic hangover of the eighties still palpable, the nineties launched with a recession that was bad enough to raise the unemployment rate, although it was an economic speed-bump compared to the soul-crushing, job-destroying Great Recession of 2008. There was a shift in the use of drugs, with people having less discretionary income to spend on recreational substances. One fashionable drug to emerge was Ecstasy, widely known as "X" or "E," an amphetamine derivative and hallucinogen that was a major part of the rave scene. Raves were peripatetic parties that featured electronic music and mind-bending light shows. Revelers would carry their own fluorescent lights, with which they'd dance frenetically to the mostly lyric-free, pulsating beats for hours on end.

"At a rave party, I saw a guy who had stuffed himself with Ecstasy repeat for hours: 'I am an orange, don't peel me, I am an orange, don't peel me,'" says Liz, a former raver. "Another guy thought he was a fly and wouldn't stop hitting his head against a window." The high, which could last up to four hours, made users feels ecstatic, joyful, exhilarated, and sensual, and it was considered the love drug of the decade. Unfortunately, X also raises body temperature and blood pressure and causes profuse sweating (possible dehydration), a racing pulse, decreased appetite, and a dry mouth. Other more serious negative side effects include heart attacks, seizures, liver damage, delirium, and coma.

X also reduces the user's awareness of the need to eat and sleep, two rather crucial elements necessary for sustaining life. "I'm lucky to be alive, but I'm still experiencing the after effects of the trauma," says the now clean and sober Liz. "Depression, anxiety, stress, recurring nightmares, and bad headaches were a few things that affected me after I took Ecstasy. I almost died. I wake up in a sweat just thanking God that it was just another nightmare. I pray that in time the nightmares will fade away." Sadly, many deaths resulted from the use of Ecstasy, but education about the drug and the disappearance of raves caused E to lose its luster.

The nineties also saw a rise in mom-and-pop meth labs and heroin use. Models like Kate Moss became the cover girls for "heroin chic," a term that glamorized the pale skin, dark-circled eyes, and emaciated figures of smack users.

The Marijuana Revolution

Marijuana is the third most popular recreational drug in America, behind only alcohol and tobacco, and it has been used by nearly a hundred million Americans. Users cut a wide swath of the population, from Gen Xers and Millennials to Boomers, as well as those who occupy the highest office in the world such as President Obama (a former member of the "Choom Gang") and the disingenuously noninhaling President Clinton.

Government surveys show that some twenty-five million Americans have smoked pot in the past year alone, with the movement to legalize cannabis for medicinal as well as recreational use receiving a groundswell of support across the country. In what seems like a head-spinning turnaround in public opinion and policy, medical marijuana is, as of this writing, legal in twenty-three states plus Washington, DC, as is recreational pot use in the states of Colorado, Oregon, and Washington. More states are waiting in the wings, watching closely to see if the tax revenues from the legal sale of pot will give our fiscally beleaguered country a much-needed boost in revenue, or if all hell will break loose. And if the momentum to legalize pot continues unabated, we might soon be washing down our fully baked goods with hemp-infused *ganjaritas* from a local cafe. What gets swept under the rug with all the media hype is that marijuana is an addictive drug that is especially damaging to young people's developing brains.

Heroin and Painkiller Epidemics

While heroin might have been the party drug of the nineties, its abuse has reached epidemic proportions in the new millennium. The number of heroin users in the United States nearly doubled between 2005 and 2012, from 380,000 to 670,000, according to a 2014 report from the National Institute on Drug Abuse. Some officials attribute the surge of smack to its low price and accessibility. In Rockland County, an affluent suburb of New York City, a bag of heroin can cost as little as five dollars and is easier for minors to buy than a six-pack of beer. Heroin use is particularly bad in New England states such as Massachusetts and Vermont, where the governors have publicly called it a state health emergency.

Equally troubling, and perhaps more insidious because of its availability via prescription pad, is opioid addiction. Among those who used illicit drugs for the first time in 2007, painkillers were one of the most popular substances— with nonmedical use rising 12 percent, according to the Foundation for a Drug-Free World. One in ten high school seniors in the United States admits to abusing prescription painkillers, with hydrocodone being the most commonly abused pharmaceutical. As drug companies made the pills harder to crush and snort or shoot up, and the FDA began to crack down on doctors who were profiting from the high demand, both teens and adults increasingly sought out the cheap, pure form of heroin readily available on the streets.

Prescription drug abuse is also climbing in older Americans, particularly abuse of the anti-anxiety drug Xanax and opioid painkiller OxyContin, while college students are using Adderall, the drug used to treat attention-deficit disorder (ADD), as a study aid. According to the health care data company IMS Health, prescription sales for stimulants increased more than fivefold between 2002 and 2012. Its off-label effect for those without ADD is to enhance concentration and learning ability, but it is also taken for the speed-like high.

Another group of recreational drugs of choice among teens and twenty-somethings are synthetics, especially bath salts, which cause a cascade of serotonin and other neurotransmitters to the brain. MDMA (methylenedioxymethamphetamine), which has the street name "Molly," is a restyled form of Ecstasy popular among the club kids today. It is said to reduce anxiety, increase feelings of connection to others, and heighten sensations. "This is a way of life for me, I've met a lot of great people, and I know it sounds weird but I've learned a lot about myself," a twenty-one-year-old who is high on Molly tells a *Boston Globe* reporter at a local club. He says he first tried Molly in 2012 and has since been showing up and glowing up at after-hours dance parties. "You're very comfortable when you are rolling," he explains, using the term for being high on Molly. "You really connect with people."

In extreme cases, Molly can cause a rapid increase in body temperature, heart rate, and blood pressure that can lead to hyperthermia and sometimes death. It has no accepted medical use and a high potential for abuse. Bootleg formulations of MDMA are being sold that contain harmful and addictive substances, fueling concerns about its safety. Around 2007, when Molly began to take off, Kanye West and Miley Cyrus started singing its praises. Today, the purer, "safer" Molly is harder to find, and therefore more young lives are at risk.

The History of Natural Highs

While people from the dawn of time have turned to alcohol and other drugs for pleasure, relief, and escape, there has always been a universal and equally powerful desire to seek pleasure without the use of mood-altering substances. In other words, people have always known that the enhanced feelings and pleasure that are caused by drugs can be produced by doing things that bring us joy and give us a sense of purpose and accomplishment. How we do this has evolved and changed over time, but as you will see, many of our natural highs remain the same, including the activities I've identified under what I'm calling the six Pleasure Principles, which will be examined further in part 2.

Yabba Dabba Do Times

Our primitive ancestors may not have gone boulder bowling like the Flinstonian vision of the Hanna-Barbera cartoon, but they did devise ways to entertain themselves through drawing, carvings, music, and other creative expressions. According to Cambridge University researchers, "finger flutings"—primitive finger painting—were discovered alongside other cave art dating back some thirteen thousand years. In New Mexico one can see thousands of petroglyphs—rock carvings of animals, the sun, and other designs—the oldest of which are from about 2000 BCE.

Anthropologists also say early humans made musical sounds with their voices between 60,000 and 30,000 BCE—around the same time they began painting and sculpting. The voice (not the TV talent show but vocal utterances) was their first musical instrument. Like prehistoric preschoolers, they made music by clapping rhythmically or hitting two stones together to create a beat. Later instruments included various types of flutes, whistles, and pipes made of wood or animal bones. Clearly, art and music were natural creative outlets that continued to evolve as we did—and in fact played a role in that evolution.

Spiritual Revitalization

Practicing Jews, Christians, and Muslims believe that people are not meant to work every day and that revitalizing one's mind, body, and spirit must involve rest, prayer, and reflection. In the book of Genesis, God, who is said to have created the universe in six days, rests on the seventh. For many Christians, Sunday is the day for prayer and reflection. For Jews, the Sabbath starts at sundown Friday and continues through Saturday. Some Orthodox Jews believe the Sabbath to be so sacred that they do not exchange money or use electricity on that day.

According to Exodus 20:10, "the seventh day is a sabbath to the Lord your God. On it you shall not do any work, neither you, nor your son or daughter, nor your male or female servant, nor your animals, nor any foreigner residing in your towns" (NIV). In Muslim countries, Friday is not a workday, and the devout are summoned to pray in a mosque. The Qur'an states: "O you who believe, when the call to prayer is made on the day of congregation, hasten to remember God, putting aside your business. This is better for you if you can understand. And when the service of prayer is over spread out in the land, and look for the bounty of God and remember God a great deal that you may prosper" (sura 62:9–10).

Meditation, which involves emptying one's mind of extraneous thoughts and experiencing the present moment, is a central part of spiritual practice in Buddhism and considered a path toward enlightenment and Nirvana (ultimate peace and contentment). In the Satipatthana Sutta, the Sanskrit discourse for establishing mindfulness, the Buddha says: "This is the direct way for the purification of beings, for the overcoming of sorrow and lamentation, for the extinguishing of suffering and grief, for walking on the path of truth, for the realization of Nirvana."

Whatever one's religion or belief system, the idea of a spiritual palate cleansing is important for the faithful and those seeking natural highs to observe.

Pagan Pleasures

Gladiators notwithstanding, the ancient Romans understood the importance of leisure activities that did not involve bacchanalias or blood sports. Activities such as swimming, horseback riding, and wrestling were a relief from a life that revolved around work and business. The Romans were a social people who enjoyed banquets, festivals, and board games (like dice, checkers, and backgammon), and who expressed their creativity through art, architecture, and theatrical performances of plays, many of which are still staged today.

Similarly, the ancient Greeks were a celebratory people who left the world their great love for sports as the creators of the Olympics, which date back to 776 BCE. The games continued for nearly twelve centuries, until Emperor Theodosius decreed in 393 CE that all such "pagan cults" be banned. But they resumed again in 1896, the official start of the modern Olympics.

Another Greek legacy borne of our natural desire to create is the theater (Dionysus was the Greek god of drama), with the first productions beginning in the sixth century BCE. The Greeks also held public festivals each year to celebrate their accomplishments and culture with dance, storytelling, and music. With thinking, learning, and debating being among Greek antiquity's greatest pleasures of the mind, it should be no surprise that the Greeks produced renowned philosophers, poets, and scholars, including Aristotle, Plato, Socrates, and Homer.

The Holiday High

Medieval entertainment in Europe varied according to one's status but included feasts, banquets, jousts, tournaments, troubadours, minstrels, jesters, acrobats, jugglers, games, and sports. Royals and peasants alike celebrated numerous holidays, such as Christmas, Easter, and May Day. On Sundays most plows came to a halt.

Like the Medievals, Elizabethans also celebrated many seasonal holidays, marked with feasts, bell ringing, dancing, and gaming. Christmas lasted through January 5. (Even back then Europeans had more vacation days.) They also found creative ways to spend their leisure time, such as singing, playing music on various instruments (including the lute, virginal, viola, recorder, bagpipe, and fiddle), and dancing. The wealthy would frequently hire musicians to play during dinner, while the townspeople would play their own music and dance at fairs and festivals. Whether it was the stately tinternell or the exuberant jig, dancing was considered a healthy recreation for the mind and exercise for the body during the Elizabethan era.

This was another period known for its theater, with productions for every class of citizen, from bawdy comedies to hanky-wringing tragedies. The first public theater in London was built in 1576, and roving troupes of all-male actors, puppeteers, and acrobats would perform across the country. Elizabethans produced some of the most brilliant playwrights of all time, including Christopher Marlow, Ben Johnson, and the immortal Bard himself, William Shakespeare. Like other periods, leisure time was also filled with games, including dice, chess, checkers, and cards, and sports such as golf, horse racing, shovelboard (a game in which pieces of metal or money are pushed on a board to reach certain marks), swimming, fishing, hunting, fencing, and cricket. It was unthinkable for a man with social clout to be unskilled at tennis, archery, or hunting.

Puritan Pleasures

The idea of Puritan pleasure sounds like an oxymoron, given the harsh, unforgiving lifestyle and strict adherence to religious observance Puritans practiced. People were fined for not attending church, for example, and confinement in stockades and public whippings were not uncommon. That said, early Americans knew how to weave some fun into their otherwise gloomy lives by singing, telling stories, and holding contests.

When children weren't helping sew, churn butter, or farm, they enjoyed playing games, including tag, hide-and-seek, hopscotch, kite flying, jump rope, London Bridge, nursery rhymes, and Blind Man's Bluff. Adults played cards when they weren't reading the Bible. And because taking a nature hike too far from the village might lead to death by wild animal or angry tribesman, a colonial family would spend a great deal of time together, gathered around the fireplace in the kitchen, which also served to keep them warm during chilly evenings.

Modern Natural High Times

The kinds of activities that Puritans engaged in for natural pleasures prevailed pretty much until the industrial revolution in the mid to late 1800s. This heralded the beginning of the modern era, when electricity, assembly line production of cars, and advances in manufacturing relieved many people of much of the drudgery of life-sustaining work and gave them the additional free time to expand their consciousness with the growing list of new entertainment and creative options (thanks in a large part to one man, Thomas Edison). That list included the telephone, phonograph, radio, motion pictures, and the ability to travel farther from home faster and more economically. The flood of immigration of people from Europe and Asia that marked this period continued to build America's image as a melting pot of different customs, music, literature, art, religion, and food that would potentially expand everyone's perspective on the variety and richness of life and human potential. Despite the horrors of two world wars and a devastating depression in between, a growing middle class laid the foundation for the prosperity of the postwar '50s that would come to define American culture—and eventually the Western world—for both good and ill.

Elizabeth, Age Eighty-Five, Retired Teacher from New York

I never drank or smoked, but when I was in college I did go to fraternity parties or to clubs in the Village where musicians smoked pot or took heroin before performing. I was a child of the Depression, so we had to make our own fun. I grew up in Sheepshead Bay, Brooklyn, so we could always hang out on the boardwalk or at the beach. It was close to Coney Island, and we'd watch the fireworks display twice a week during the summer. We also spent a lot of time playing stoop ball, stick ball, and a game called kick the can, which was like hide-and-seek. We'd play and dance the Lindy in the middle of the street. We just loved to dance!

My girlfriends and I decided to start a library, gathering books from our parents and bringing them to someone's house where kids could borrow any book. There were public libraries, of course, but we thought it would be a fun thing to do. I remember one paperback novel called *The Impatient Virgin*, which disappeared immediately, much to our amusement. We never knew what happened to that book.

During hot summer days, we'd see a double feature at the cinema, which was the only place that was air conditioned. It cost twenty-five cents. My mother and I would go for a weekend to the Catskills (we couldn't afford to stay longer than that), where we'd swim, eat, play sports, and watch the Borscht Belt comedians. It was the highlight of my year!

Going to the movies was one of our major sources of entertainment during the '40s. We had big movie stars like Clark Gable, Tyrone Power, Gary Cooper, Frank Sinatra, Greta Garbo, and Bette Davis. We'd also sometimes go to the drugstore, which, at that time, served ice cream soda at the counter for twenty-five cents.

Radio was huge back then. We'd gather around the radio as a family to listen to soap operas. There were mysteries like *The Shadow*, and comedies like Burns and Allen, Jack Benny, Eddie Cantor. That was our family entertainment. I got my own radio and phonograph for my birthday, which was fantastic. Nothing was expensive at the time because no one had any money, at least in my neighborhood.

Hipsters and Hippies

Despite the looming threat of the Cold War and Vietnam, the fifties and sixties was a time of unbridled optimism, which included men walking on the moon. The youth culture unleashed a barrage of movements—feminism, civil rights, anti-establishment, and, of course, anti-war. Folk singers and Flower Children participated in protest marches, sit-ins, moratoriums, rock concerts, and rallies. Kids growing up during this time watched TV—a lot of it—some of it in living color.

Poodle skirts, miniskirts, Nehru shirts, pop artists like Andy Warhol, and an outpouring of musical talent from Motown and Bob Dylan to the Rolling Stones and the Beatles all drew from the belief that times were changing—for the better. Although the Beatles, like many musicians, experimented with drugs and influenced a generation to follow suit, they also traveled to India in 1968 to attend a Transcendental Meditation training session with Maharishi Mahesh Yogi. Their interest in the Maharishi changed people's attitudes about spirituality and encouraged the study of Transcendental Meditation in the West. This was one example of the great expansion of interest in Eastern religions, including Buddhism, Hinduism, and Taoism, as people sought meaning beyond drugs and Western religious ideas.

Women enjoyed a newfound status in the workforce, delaying or forgoing marriage for a career, and using birth control pills in record numbers (ten million by 1973) to have sex for pleasure rather than procreation. Gay, lesbian, bisexual, and transgender people, who were beginning to emerge from the closet, also enjoyed a pre-AIDS period of sexual freedom and exuberance.

TV shows like *The Brady Bunch*, with its blended family, *The Mary Tyler Moore Show*, with its "single girl" lifestyle, and *All in the Family*, with its exposed political incorrectness, all held mirrors to our popular culture, which was becoming, in many ways, more sophisticated in showing an expanded consciousness of human rights and potential. The civil rights and feminist marches in the sixties also brought more people to the streets to celebrate equality rather than turning on and dropping out.

**Lenny, Age Thirty-Nine,
Fundraiser from Florida**

I was really into science fiction in the seventies. I went
to this arts camp when I was thirteen, where I hung
out with a group of guitarists, all of whom were into
Star Trek. I hadn't even heard of *Star Trek* at the time,
but I wanted to be part of the group, so I watched
all the shows and read as much as I could about it.
I remember going together to a *Star Trek* convention,
where I wore Spock ears. It was one of the first trips
I took by myself to meet my friends. My obsession
lasted until I went to college, and we all ended up at
Princeton. I realize it seems nerdy, but I never did any
drugs or alcohol. I had fun bonding with others over
a mutual interest. It doesn't matter what your hobby
is—in my case it was *Star Trek*—it feels great to be
a part of a community, which has its own culture.
I think that's what drugs are all about for some
people. There's peer pressure to get involved and
a sense of community and a shared experience,
especially for young people.

The Boom and Crash

The '80s was another period marked by optimism about the
future. But instead of eschewing the establishment, young
people with degrees from elite colleges and fresh out of
business school vied for six-figure salaries. Men wore gar-
ish sweaters, and women sported big hair and linebacker
shoulder pads for their hundred-yard career fast track. The
Internet was still a twinkle in Bill Gates's eye, so people
entertained themselves with VCRs, boom boxes, Pac-Man,
Rubik's Cubes, Trivial Pursuit, flashdancing, going for
the burn with Jane Fonda, and MTV (in the days before
iTunes, everyone wanted their MTV). Cheesy pop music was

mixed with hits from megastars like Michael Jackson and Madonna.

While the eighties and nineties seemed to be a time of greed and the superficial pleasures of pop culture, people around the world had the same universal yearnings for meaning and authentic joy as humans have had throughout history. For one thing, this was a period when, despite the backsliding during the Reagan years, consciousness of our dependence on and identification with the natural world had quietly begun to grow and inspire people at the grassroots level to begin to do something about climate change and the mass extinction of species. This found expression eventually in the local and national movements that continue to blossom today. For many people this was an opportunity to expand their consciousness beyond the addictive consumer mentality and to see themselves as a part of something bigger than their egoistic striving for status and wealth.

Getting High Tech

The World Wide Web was born in 1992 and would forever change the way we communicate and socialize, spend our money, do business, and entertain and educate ourselves. Although the world didn't come to a halt after Y2K (the turn of the century when computers across the world were supposed to crash simultaneously), we would suffer a permanent loss of innocence after 9/11, two devastating wars, and a recession from which we have yet to fully recover. But the new millennium also ushered in a new technological revolution that gave us smartphones, YouTube, Twitter, Facebook, Instagram, apps, blogs, and texts, all of which take up countless hours of our leisure time and enable us to connect with a larger group of friends (and strangers).

Many people own a smartphone—a portable computer and camera that enables them to communicate with others on a nearly constant basis, upload media, and get instant news flashes with the touch of a screen or the flick of their thumb. And while some bemoan the loss of the simple pleasures of the past, technology has produced a wide range of new creative outlets for citizen journalists, photographers, cooks, directors, podcasters, bloggers, vloggers, and self-published authors. All of this posting and sharing is part of an expanded socialization universe, which can potentially open our minds and our borders and bring us closer together by expanding our consciousness beyond the boundaries of any LSD trip. At the same time there is concern that our compulsive use of these devices is like an addiction that can cut us off from authentic relationships in the real world.

This partial tour of humanity's search for something beyond the ordinary—for pleasure, for meaning—doesn't do justice to the complexity and significance of this unending quest. Can we ever find the source and purpose of this mysterious need to be high? Some say it all begins—and ends—in our brains.

2

The Craving Brain

"I Need, I Need!"

What part does our brain play in our desire to relieve pain, stress, or depression, or simply to seek pleasure? And given our natural craving to get high, why are some people satisfied by natural pleasures and can take or leave alcohol and other drugs, while others can't get enough? Some of the answers can be found in the research currently being done on substance abuse, which shows addiction and alcoholism to be a brain disease with some genetic components. It seems our desire to get high, whether through mood-altering substances or natural, healthier activities that bring pleasure, is all controlled by the brain—the captain, if you will, of the ship that is our body.

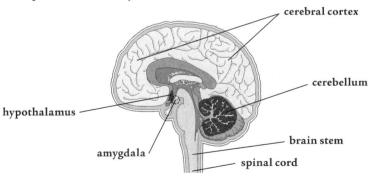

How the Brain Works

Despite all the research and the development of neuroimaging technology, scientists are still mystified by what goes on between our ears. But here are a few basics facts that we do know.

The adult brain weighs about three pounds and is a combination of flesh, nerves, and fluid. It looks a bit like a walnut but is soft to the touch. It contains a billion or so specialized cells called neurons that communicate and form networks via chemicals called neurotransmitters and electrical charges that pass through the tiny gaps, or synapses, between the neurons. Every part of our brain serves a different function, but the simplest way to understand how our brain works is to think about it as having three parts: primitive, emotional, and thinking.

The Primitive Brain

The brain stem sits on top of the spine and is in charge of our automatic functions, like breathing, heartbeat, digestion, reflexes, sleep, and arousal. The spinal cord is the messenger that communicates with the rest of our body, and the cerebellum (not to be confused with something from the pre-Civil War era) regulates our balance and coordination, which are necessary for doing things like riding a bike and catching a ball. If you are always the last to be picked for a sports team, you can blame your cerebellum.

Our brain is also divided into two hemispheres: right and left. They are similar but not identical, and are connected by a thick band of fibers and nerves. Each side functions slightly differently from the other one. Even neuroscientists don't fully understand why the messages sent from the two hemispheres to the rest of our body crisscross, so the right side controls our left side and vice versa. Every brain is unique, and if you know which side of your brain is weaker, you can exercise it the way you do your muscles. You can strengthen and repair your brain by making new neurons—more on that later.

The two hemispheres work as a unit rather than as two independent systems, but there are some differences. The left brain is responsible for language and serves as our analytical and logical side; the right hemisphere is home to our visual and spatial ability. It sees the larger picture and recognizes faces, and it is stimulated by artistic and musical activities, as well as our emotional perceptions. Some believe it is also where our sense of humor resides.

The Emotional Brain

Also known as our limbic system, the emotional brain is located deep inside the midbrain and acts as the gatekeeper between the spinal cord and the thinking brain in the cerebrum, which sits above it. It regulates our survival instincts, including sex drive, sleep cycle, and hunger, as well as our emotions, fear, sensory perceptions (vision, hearing, touch, smell, taste), and pleasure. The so-called pleasure center or reward circuit is also based in the limbic system, so thrill seekers can thank this part of the brain for fueling many of their cravings and desires.

The limbic system includes the amygdala, which is responsible for determining which memories are stored in the brain and where. It is believed what we remember is based on how big an emotional response an event invokes (important, frightening, or enjoyable events are filed in our long-term memory). The limbic system also incorporates the hypothalamus, which controls our biological clock and hormones, and the thalamus, which passes sensory information to the thinking centers in our cortex.

The Thinking Brain

The cerebral cortex consists of the sensory, motor, and association areas; it is the thinking part of our brain and is often considered the crown jewel of our body, as it sits on top and controls our thoughts, reasoning, language, planning, and imagination. Voluntary movement, vision, hearing, speech, and judgment reside here as well. This part of the brain is not fully developed until our mid-twenties, which is why teenagers are more susceptible to risk-taking behavior, including abusing drugs and alcohol. Binging and overindulging in any mood-altering substances can prevent the brain from properly forming.

"A teen is especially prone to addiction," said Amir Levine, a Columbia University psychiatrist and neuroscientist who spoke at the 2014 World Science Festival symposium on addiction and the brain. This is particularly true of teens who smoke cigarettes. "Our studies have shown that the majority of cocaine users start as cigarette smokers, and nicotine also makes someone more susceptible to drug use by changing the DNA in their brain. This continues up to the age 25." Levine added that, contrary to popular belief, nicotine is a gateway drug to the harder stuff, including cocaine.

Your Brain on Drugs

Psychoactive drugs, including amphetamines, barbiturates, nicotine, opioids, and hallucinogens, tap into the brain's communication system by disrupting the way nerve cells normally send, receive, and process information. There are several ways drugs are able to do this, including overstimulating the pleasure center or reward circuit of the brain.

Marc Lewis, a neuroscientist and professor of psychology at Radboud University in Holland, is a recovering drug addict. His rap sheet of substances includes opiates, opium, nitrous oxide, pot, and alcohol. In 2006, Lewis quit drugs for good and began studying the brain changes that intensify cravings and weaken our self-control. His book, *Memoirs of an Addicted Brain*, combines his personal story with an account of how drugs and addiction seriously alter the brain's neural chemistry and structure.

It works something like this: dopamine is a hormone released by the brain whenever we pursue something that we crave. As Levine explained to the audience at the World Science Festival: "Dopamine is absorbed by brain structures responsible for narrowed attention, effortful action and, above all, desire—the visceral thrust that motivates goal seeking. When addiction sets in—whether to drugs, booze, cigarettes, sex, gambling, food, or something else— what starts out as an episode of pleasure (or relief) begins to control the dopamine pump." It should be noted that the "narrowed attention, effortful action, and . . . desire" associated with intense exercise and other activities under the umbrella of our six Pleasure Principles also produces dopamine. (More about that later.)

For addicts, Lewis says, the release of dopamine is followed by the anticipation of getting more, and the neural networks of desire become increasingly focused on that goal. Those networks also become desensitized to other, healthier goals, such as enjoying work, spending time with family and friends, and self-preservation. When addicts feel a sense of excitement at the thought of getting whatever substance they desire, their brain craving intensifies. As this cycle repeats, areas of the cortex—the part of the brain that represents what's important and valuable—gets rewired.

Lewis experienced this recircuiting of his brain, which blocked out his healthier instincts and led him to engage in criminal activities, including stealing morphine from labs where he worked and breaking into pharmacies to get his fixes. As Lewis's story illustrates, drugs do not discriminate. Neurologically speaking, whether one is book smart or street smart, an addict's synapses become laser-focused on thinking, reminiscing, planning, and imagining ways to get high.

For those who study addiction, the concept of cravings comes up often. Researchers believe that cravings are also a response to memories of the drug experience. Our brain remembers what is pleasurable and what is not, so the intense neurotransmitter release that comes with taking drugs is responsible for our brain's creating lasting memories that spark our cravings. MRIs (magnetic resonance images) show intense activity in the brains of addicts when they view pictures of things associated with drug use (such as a crack pipe or white powdery substances resembling heroin or cocaine).

In the act of remembering the brain reexperiences an event, so reliving a drug experience will cause an emotional reaction. While we are recalling something, cortical areas associated with the sights, sounds, smells, and thoughts related to the event are also activated, and we want to relive that initial experience. This is why a smoldering cigarette might trigger someone to want a drink, if they associate smoking with alcohol.

Your Brain on Alcohol

Alcoholics can do as much damage to their brains (and other vital organs) as people can do with drugs. Once alcohol enters the bloodstream, every organ, including the liver, the heart, and the brain, will be negatively affected. If you are a blackout drunk, the brain drain will cause you to suffer even worse. The brain, which needs a constant blood supply, is particularly vulnerable to the effects of alcohol.

Most alcoholics have some loss of mental function, reduced brain size, and changes in the function of brain cells.

Research suggests that women are more vulnerable than men to alcohol-induced brain damage. To a much lesser degree, beer, red wine, and vermouth can trigger migraines, especially in women who are prone to these types of headaches. If a woman drinks while pregnant, she also risks causing neural damage to her child. Fetal Alcohol Syndrome (FAS) can produce developmental delays, poor motor skills, lack of concentration, and myriad behavioral problems, including hyperactivity and mental and social anxiety.

And if you think you are different because you can "hold your liquor," think again. Research shows that those who are able to drink large amounts of alcohol in one sitting without getting sloppy drunk are at a higher, not lower, risk of developing an addiction. This is why one should never engage in a chugging contest or try to drink someone "under the table." Chances are you will end up on top of an examining table in the emergency room instead.

Of course, no one takes that first drink intending to become an alcoholic, but developing a high tolerance for liquor is one way to get there. Here's a common trajectory: You've had a stressful day, so you pour yourself a glass of wine or beer to take the edge off. The next time you feel stressed, you remember how much better you felt after that drink, so you have another stress-relieving nip. The problem is that, if you're an alcoholic, your body will need more and more liquor to get the same pleasurable feeling. This is what's known as "tissue tolerance." Tissue tolerance happens with drugs as well, and one can also build up a resistance to over-the-counter medications, including sleep aids, allergy medicine, and prescription painkillers. Our body's tissue tolerance is what sets the wheels of alcoholism and drug addiction in motion. The more addicts use a substance, the more their bodies will need so that it can work its magic.

Brain Cravings

Addiction experts say that the powerful craving for drugs can linger months or years after a recovering addict quits, and this can lead to a relapse. After a long period of use, the addict or alcoholic no longer uses to get high (the initial goal) but in order to feel normal. "Drugs damage the part of the brain responsible for willpower," explains Eric Nestler, a neuroscientist and professor of psychiatry at New York's Mount Sinai School of Medicine, who spoke at the 2014 World Science Festival. "It's similar to not being able to put on the brakes even though your car is headed straight into a tree."

Scientists have discovered that this chemical craving is due in part to long-term changes in brain function. It is a conditioned response to powerful cues to use, such as people, places, and things associated with alcohol or other drugs. These memories of getting high can trigger the reward system in the brain that produces irresistible urges. Think about your most vivid memories. If we experience something that is unpleasant, like a death in the family, illness, pain, or humiliation, we are more likely to remember it. It's the same for rewarding experiences, such as the birth of a child, a wedding, a fun vacation, or an intense high. When positive things happen, MRIs show that the part of our brain associated with rewards lights up like a Christmas tree. This chemical reaction is why those in recovery should avoid evoking these emotional memories and steer clear of friends or places they associate with using. Similarly, when a person undergoes stress, such as job loss, these negative experiences make a user vulnerable to relapse. Part of the recovery process is learning how to deal with these triggers and cravings. What I've been describing about the how the brain processes drug cravings also applies to food, gambling, sex, and other so-called process addictions as well.

"The brain is constantly remodeling itself," said Nora Volkow, director of the National Institute on Drug Abuse at the National Institutes of Health as well as a panelist at the World Science Festival. "Drugs increase the dopamine, which stimulates the memories that stay with you for years after drug use stops. This is why it is so easy to relapse."

The good news, however, is that our brains can recover even from years of abuse because they have a reparative ability called neuroplasticity, which involves producing new brain cells. The time it takes to repair the brain depends on an individual's health and age. A twenty-something's brain, for example, will bounce back more quickly than that of a fifty-something who has been using for decades. This ability to regenerate new synapses has been shown to be a key factor in recovery from addiction. As addicts change their behavior using the recovery tools they learn in treatment and in Twelve Step programs such as Alcoholics Anonymous (AA) and Narcotics Anonymous (NA), their brains actually change so that cravings decrease and dopamine and other feel-good chemicals are generated by the positive feelings that come with the rewards of recovery activities. These include the recovering addict learning to practice the six Pleasure Principles I'll cover in part 2.

Brain Boosters

Neuroenhancing stimulants such as Adderall and Ritalin, originally prescribed for children and adults with ADD and attention-deficit/hyperactivity disorder (ADHD), are now being used by tens of thousands of college students seeking "steroids" for the brain. These drugs are not just used recreationally or to enhance one's senses but to get a competitive edge.

A warning to those who are toying with the idea of taking a "smart" pill: While juicing the brain will improve your ability to focus and recall data (temporarily), it will not make you more intelligent, nor is it safe. No one knows yet what the long-term effects of these drugs will be, and there have been many cases of young people who get addicted. We do know that these drugs activate the brain's reward pathways, which are part of the neural circuitry that controls mood. Human and animal studies have shown that taking these medications could alter the brain's structure and function in ways that produce depression, anxiety, and cognitive decline. There have also been numerous cases of drug-induced psychosis and even suicides.

Treating the Craving Bain

Because drugs and alcohol change the very fabric of our brain structure, the path to "curing" addiction, if such a thing is possible, has never been easy. Like people with other diseases, experts say, most users do not have the ability to stop without some kind of intervention, be it AA, rehabilitation, or individual or group therapy. Yet scientists are continuing to search for a viable medical option that could help defuse the cravings without replacing one addictive drug with another, as is the case with methadone.

Several new treatments for tricking the brain or blocking messages have already been developed. Daniela Schiller, an assistant professor of neuroscience and psychiatry at Mount Sinai School of Medicine, is working with others on a drug that will help humans forget certain memories, including traumas and pleasurable feelings one gets when using.

Schiller has studied the use of a common beta blocker that latches onto receptors in a variety of proteins that interfere with the formation of memories. This process is called memory reconsolidation, and it allows competing memories to become one. Reconsolidation might be a promising treatment for drug addiction because people can't get addicted to a pleasurable experience if they don't recall it. By comparison, behavior therapies for addiction often fail, and relapses are common. Schiller's studies have demonstrated that we might be able to eliminate some of our most stressful memories by zapping them at just the right time.

Unlike with electroshock therapy, which sometimes results in memory loss, the patient produces a different memory without the emotional component that fuels the desire for drugs. "The biggest problem for most addicts is how to deal with relapse," Schiller told a reporter from the *New Yorker* in 2014. "Let's say somebody is drug free and then goes and hangs out with friends at a park. He might see a cue associated with his drug use, and that will induce a craving that will cause him to seek the drug. Reconsolidation gives the addict an opportunity to disrupt that process, where the memory isn't lost, but the pleasant feelings associated with it are gone."

Other antidotes now being used include a life-saving emergency drug called naloxone, which is also known by the brand name Narcan. It has reversed tens of thousands of drug overdoses by blocking hormone receptors from receiving the opiate, saving thousands of lives, according to a new study from the Centers for Disease Control and Prevention (CDC). In under a minute, naloxone, which is administered by injection, stops an overdose on opiates and helps restore regular breathing and consciousness in someone who has overdosed on heroin. One dose typically costs two dollars.

Because it is an opiate antagonist, it's not effective in stopping an overdose on cocaine, alcohol, or sedatives.

First approved by the FDA in the seventies, naloxone was used only in emergency rooms and ambulances. But thanks to community-based programs, the drug has seen wider distribution in fifteen states and Washington, DC. Thousands of fatal overdoses occur every year, and this drug has reduced deaths when people are given information, training, and tools to administer naloxone in emergency situations. Sharon Stancliff, the medical director of the Harm Reduction Coalition, wants naloxone to be sold over the counter. *Time* magazine explains why: "The drug is safe and non-addictive and it cannot be misused (indeed, it blocks the action of opioids, so it produces the opposite of a high), and so the more places it is available, the more likely that it will be within reach when needed." To further curtail overdoses, Stancliff says more states could pass what are called Good Samaritan laws, which give amnesty to people who call 911 and report a drug overdose.

Even better than nalaxone would be an available drug that prevents an overdose from happening in the first place. Kim Janda, professor of chemistry at the Scripps Research Institute, has helped create such a vaccine to treat heroin addiction by preventing the pleasurable effects of the drug from reaching the brain. Unfortunately, he and his colleagues have been unable to find a pharmaceutical company willing to finance and produce it. Janda says companies have summarily turned him down because the vaccine can't be manufactured cheaply enough for people to afford it. Even the government, still entrenched in the unwinnable war on drugs, is not willing to finance the vaccine. "Politicians believe that addiction is a moral failure not a disease," says Janda, "so they have less incentive to put money into treatment."

Natural Highs
Versus Chemical Highs

It is a universal truth that we all experience pain and anxiety at some point in our lives. (If you haven't, please share your story with the rest of the class.) So why are some people who have similar problems and triggers for drug use able to soothe themselves with natural highs while others self-medicate? "When we have dinner with friends, have sex, exercise, or have fun, it releases dopamine in our brain, which is our chemical reward system," explains Nestler, the neuroscientist at Mount Sinai School of Medicine. "Addicts lose the ability to feel good without drugs or alcohol, but these natural rewards are our strongest highs."

There's evidence coming out of peer addiction recovery groups that several risk and resilience factors can predict who will misuse drugs and who will instead seek natural highs from the kinds of activities noted by Nestler. Risk factors include poverty; friends who use; accessibility to drugs, which can include wealthy users with the means to finance their addictions; parents who use, are absent, or neglectful; and unemployment. Red flags include smoking at an early age, early sexual activity, stress, depression, and positive feelings when taking drugs.

We can develop resilience, however, by having positive role models, the support of family and peers, economic stability, no loss or separation issues as a child, a good relationship with parents and other family members, strong religious or moral values, high self-esteem, and a commitment to education.

Part 2 of this book has suggestions for how to experience some natural highs and reduce the risk of misusing drugs. Start feeding the reward center of your craving brain, and fill it with as many enjoyable, long-term memories as possible!

3

Birds Do It, Bees Do It

The Biology of the Buzz

Giorgio Samorini, who studies the use of plants among humans and animals, found that taking drugs is part of a universal, biologically based drive to alter consciousness. In his book *Animals and Psychedelics* Samorini explores this phenomenon and concludes that animals, like humans, deliberately get high. Rejecting the Western cultural assumption that drug use is unnatural, Samorini goes even further by exploring the possibility that use of psychedelics can create new patterns of behavior that might change a species as it evolves over time.

Based in part on Samorini's extensive research on animal use of psychoactive substances, and combined with the work of Ronald K. Siegel, a professor of psychiatry and biobehavioral sciences at the University of California, Los Angeles, the following menagerie of animal ways to escape the ordinary—both chemically and naturally—demonstrates that the need to get high is indeed universal and that our six Pleasure Principles apply across species.

High-Low Kitty

Most cat owners are familiar with the effects of catnip on their pets, which have helped spawn a hugely profitable animal toy industry as well as countless viral videos. The feline-friendly herb (*Nepeta cataria*), which is a member of the mint family, can turn the most apathetic couch potato into a furry ball of ecstasy. The most ardent nipper will react to the smell by rolling, flipping, rubbing, and sometimes drooling. When eaten, however, catnip seems to have the opposite effect, mellowing most cats out. Scientists aren't sure what the neurological explanation is for this high-low kitty reaction, but it's thought that catnip stimulates the receptors in the brain that respond to feel-good pheromones.

Catnip can also be an aphrodisiac for some cats. When taken in concentrated doses, males get erections; females adopt mating stances, complete with catcalling, come-hither vocalizations, and "love biting" of any available object if not partnered with a tomcat. Call it *50 Shades of Blue-Grays*.

The effects of catnip (which is not addictive) usually last only around ten minutes, after which the cat will lose interest and probably need a two-hour nap before becoming susceptible to catnip again. Not all cats are nip-crazy; sensitivity to the herb is inherited, and young kittens are immune to its charms. Domesticated cats are becoming increasingly unresponsive to its allure: current studies show that only 50 to 70 percent of indoor cats respond to catnip, which some researchers think may be an evolutionary adaptation after generations of having little or no contact with the actual plant. Others believe that the lack of response to catnip has more to do with a particular gene not present in all cats.

Anecdotally, my own cats not only are catnip fanciers but have a similar reaction to valerian, the herbal supplement that induces relaxation in humans. Their reaction to the smell mimics their reaction to catnip, including the head rubbing and goofy playfulness. There have been reports of catatonic reactions to valerian and other plants, the earliest of which, written by Dr. Raffaele Valieri of Naples, appeared in the 1800s: "When a sack of valerian is scattered on the earth, it is a curious and enjoyable spectacle to watch cats approach it: they roll on top of it, inhale it repeatedly, and finally begin to tremble, their fur standing on end, then leap about disjointedly, making a thousand dancing gestures of unbridled, drunken bliss, and finally losing their senses and falling into a doze, remaining excited and dazed for a long time."

The euphoria experienced by Western felines high on catnip and valerian appears tame compared to what happens when Japanese cats eat a plant called *matatabi*. "After chewing its leaves," Samorini writes, "the cats stretch out on their backs with their paws up and remain motionless in this position for some time, in apparent or perhaps real ecstasy." One might argue that it is difficult to tell whether these cats are experiencing a euphoric reaction or simply doing what they do best—sleeping—and perhaps having a wonderful dream.

Feline Fun: Natural Highs

Catnip and valerian are not the only ways for a domesticated kitty to have fun. Purring, which is one of the most obvious ways to tell that a cat is content, begins when a kitten is suckling and continues throughout its life when being stroked or snuggling next to a furry or human companion. Cats will knead a lap or blanket and sometimes salivate when they are fully grown, as they recall that pleasurable memory of being fed by their mother. Cats also enjoy hunting, stalking prey (real or imagined), chasing, curling up in small spaces, scratching, and, of course, sleeping about twenty hours a day.

They will actually feel depressed, bored, or like an irritated teen when deprived of these pleasurable instincts. Watching birds, squirrels, and other wildlife provides them with visual pleasure, and jumping, climbing, and scratching give them physical pleasure. If you have an indoor cat, you can pop in a DVD or use a cat app to see if they start tracking the motions of the other animals or swatting the screen. Computer screen savers with flapping butterflies, scurrying mice, burbling fish, or bouncing balls can also act as substitutes for the real thing. If left to their own (not electronic) devices, two cats will stalk each other and play-fight, tumbling over one another like furry competitors in the World Wrestling Federation.

Play Like a Dog: Natural Highs

As anyone from the forty-three million American dog-owning households will tell you, dogs are among the most loyal, fun-loving, playful pets. They enjoy playing fetch, catch (balls or Frisbees), and tug-of-war, as well as other games. And while human interaction is much desired, dogs also need to socialize with other canines because, try as we do, we cannot provide the same type of pleasure they get from members of their own species. As pack animals, dogs form strong bonds to each other through primal, hierarchical play. This includes chasing, sniffing, playful nipping (as opposed to aggressive biting), and mounting, which are attempts to show dominance. These activities, in addition to a loving, caring, and nurturing person or family who will tend to their needs for food, shelter, grooming, and love, reflect several of the Pleasure Principles we'll be exploring in part 2.

CANE-TOADY CANINES

Dog owners in Queensland, Australia, should beware of cane toads, which are common in this region and excrete a toxin in their sweat that is poisonous to dogs. By licking a toad, a dog can ingest enough of the toxin for it to cause profuse salivation, shaking, vomiting, and even death. Still, like four-legged street junkies, these cane toad–loving canines keep coming back for more. While an addiction to cane toads may seem like a stretch, Jonathon Cochrane of the University of Queensland's School of Veterinary Science said he treats dogs for cane toad poisoning a few times a year.

An Elephant Walked into a Bar . . .

The inebriated elephant, unlike lesser-known last-calls of the wild, is a well-known phenomenon. African elephants enjoy a variety of fruits, including those from doum, marula, mgongo, and palmyra trees, all of which are not available at your local produce stand or supermarket. The elephants will eat these fermented fruits whether scattered on the ground or shaken from the tree by their trunks or enormous bodies. The fermentation of fruits produces ethyl alcohol that can be as high as 7 percent, and when the juice enters the animal's digestive tract, even higher levels of alcohol get absorbed into their system. Researchers have seen herds of elephants appear to compete for these fruits, racing one another in an attempt to consume the most in the shortest amount of time. This pursuit of drunken pleasure is clearly not accidental but intentional. While herds usually roam no more than six miles through the forest on any given day, when these palm fruits ripen, adult males have been known to wander away from the herd and cover more than twenty miles a day in order to reach the trees bearing the fruit. As elephants famously possess good memories, there is no need for a GPS to find the exact location of these makeshift arbor saloons.

Elephant mothers, which feed their calves by letting them put their trunks inside their mouths, will unwittingly pass on the taste for the intoxicating fruit to their young. Calves not only get drunk from their mother's fruit, they learn to appreciate and seek it out again in order to get high.

How, you might wonder, does an inebriated elephant behave? Like bad drunks, some elephants can react defensively or become aggressive. It might seem like a no-brainer, but author Samorini warns those on safaris to assiduously avoid a herd of drunken elephants, as they are considered to be dangerous. (And the same might be said of a polluted pack of burly tailgaters at a football game.)

OTHER FRUIT FLIES

Elephants are one of several species that eagerly seek out fermented fruit, especially durian. Others known to enjoy fruit cocktails from time to time include orangutans, squirrels, fruit bats, and Sumatran tigers. Since tigers are avid carnivores, scientists are not certain if they like the durian for its intoxicating effect or for its taste. But the native people of Sumatra have reported cases where children carrying baskets of durian back to their village have been attacked by tigers, not to feast off their human flesh, but rather to pilfer the fruits of their labor.

Pachyderm Pleasures: Natural Highs

While elephants, like people, sometimes belly up to the fruit bar, they are primarily known as social animals that live in family groups. And when it comes to relationships, it seems some elephants never forget. The Asian variety remember old pals and have larger social networks of friends than scientists previously thought, studies have shown. Just like humans, some elephants are social butterflies, while others prefer to stick to a close-knit group of friends. Dr. Shermin de Silva from the University of Pennsylvania, who studied elephants in Sri Lanka, said, "Elephants are able to track one another over large distances by calling to each other and using their sense of smell. Our work shows that they are able to recognize their friends and renew these bonds even after being apart for a long time."

Elephants are deeply emotional and intelligent creatures that exhibit love, compassion, and grief. From the time a baby elephant is born, it immediately bonds with and receives love from its mother and other female herd members, which tend to the calf. The young elephant spends its early years being snuggled, caressed, and guided by the females (cows). If a calf is in danger, its mother will risk her own life to save her baby. If a mother dies, another cow will adopt and nurture the baby. Elderly females are closely involved with babies until they reach their teen years, when they no longer need supervision. (You may say "awww" aloud here.)

This compassionate society, in which animals express their love for one another, could be a model for humans. If one member of the herd is infirm, for example, other, stronger elephants help and care for it. They may use their trunks to massage the weak elephant's shoulders and head. They also use their trunks to prod sick elephants to their feet, and their bodies to support that of an injured or sick elephant Apparently, in the pachyderm world, it does indeed take a village.

Flipper Flips Out

Dolphins, arguably one of the smartest creatures in the animal kingdom, have discovered a way to get high by huffing

puffer fish. It seems these round, porcupine-like sea creatures release nerve toxins when provoked that can produce
a narcotic effect. Underwater footage from a BBC documentary shows young dolphins inhaling the toxins and then
passing the fish to other dolphins like loose joints.

Rob Pilley, a zoologist and producer of the series,
explained that it was "a case of young dolphins purposely
experimenting with something we know to be intoxicating," much like thrill-seeking teenagers. "After chewing
the puffer gently and passing it around, they began acting
most peculiarly, "hanging around with their noses at the
surface as if fascinated by their own reflection." Similar
to the trippy cane toads, inhaling too much of the puffer
fish (also coincidentally known as blowfish) can be deadly
to dolphins, and a low dose can trigger a trance-like state,
causing Flipper to flip out.

Pods of Fun: Natural Highs

Dolphins are so intelligent that these mammals invent new
games to entertain themselves throughout their lives. In
fact, dolphins spend a good portion of each day playing.
Depending on the pod, dolphins create different types of
games and playful behaviors, which do not include performing at the pleasure of spectators at Sea World. That's
called work.

They are agile swimmers, of course, and enjoy leaping
out of the water and doing somersaults in the air. They
also enjoy body surfing and have been seen catching a wave
alongside boarders, as well as swimming in the bow waves
produced by boats.

Curious dolphins also find pleasure playing with sea-
weed, coral, fish, and trash, or anything else they find floating in the deep. They have even been observed in the wild
playing games of catch and frolicking with fish and other

mammals in the ocean. Dolphins often chase one another or challenge their porpoise pals to speed races that can last for hours.

On some occasions, dolphins in the wild will play with the people who share their surf turf by jumping over kayaks, poking scuba divers, or splashing swimmers—all of which is just good fin fun.

Like elephants, they also find pleasure in familial and social bonding and traveling in pods of up to twelve animals, and they can display altruism, sacrificing their own well-being to care for injured or sick family and pod members. There are also stories of dolphins rescuing humans who are in distress at sea, which unfortunately has led to their exploitation by ocean theme parks and the military.

Crazy Horse

A popular drug among horses, mules, donkeys, cows, sheep, antelopes, pigs, and rabbits is the appropriately named locoweed, a type of legume also called crazy grass or crazy seeds that acts as a mind-altering drug. Unfortunately, locoweed is to these animals what meth is to people: an addictive drug that can kill them over the course of time. During the lean winter months, locoweed is the only green plant available in some pastures, so grazers often eat it initially as a food source and then return frequently for its psychoactive effects. Because the weed is so dangerous to herds, ranchers are constantly on guard for signs of locoweed abuse, but the plant is abundant in certain regions and virtually impossible to fully eradicate.

One of the earliest reported cases of locoism occurred in 1873, when Californian horses and cows were observed behaving peculiarly in their pastures. It seems the animals were able to distinguish the intoxicating grass from the purely nutritional kind and habitually sought out and devoured locoweed. Sadly, the sins of the mothers are often passed to the children. Foals and calves following their mom's lead will also seek out the intoxicating plant and become young addicts.

In 1883, farmers in Kansas spoke of the crazy grass epidemic, in which twenty-five thousand cows went on a normal grass fast, determined instead to search for locoweed. Loco fever reached herds in Mexico, Arizona, and the loony and lonely prairies of Montana. The side effects caused by locoweed addiction include a serious case of paranoia. Animals would be found hiding behind boulders or among camouflaging trees. In some cases, their eyes would be fixed and bulging, or they would be lie prostrate on the ground in a state of advanced intoxication.

Many farmers were forced to abandon their pastures after a locoweed infestation that nearly wiped out all other grasses. Some scientists suspect this untapped growth might have been caused by the scattering of seeds by whacked-out cattle and horses. The addiction was so great that animals would tear through sacks containing the grass and overturn wagons where it was stashed. Unfortunately, many of these crack horses starved themselves to death in their single-minded quest to get high.

Horse Play: Natural Highs

There are several types of equine entertainment, especially among those that have space to roam. Horses enjoy nuzzling and pushing objects, such as balls, as well as play-fighting and sexual play, especially with other young horses. They will gallop across a field for no apparent reason or buck in an exuberant release of energy. As with all animals that typically live in groups, the ability to run freely and socialize with other horses provides an opportunity for them to engage in playful and pleasurable behavior.

Big Horny Sheep

In the vast wilderness of the Canadian Rockies lives a unique species of yellow-green lichen. Despite the fact that it contains no nutritional value, bighorn sheep that get a whiff of the lichen will risk life and cloven hoof to score some. Once they reach a lichen, the animals will rub their teeth down to the gums in order to scrape off every last bit of it. Fortunately, these narcotic lichens are rare and only grow in some desolate parts of the Rockies, making it difficult for them to form a cartel.

Sheepish Behavior: Natural Highs

Healthy lambs are usually very active, and group play is common. They love to climb and are curious about their surroundings. Like most adolescents, as lambs get older, they spend less time with their mothers and more time with their peers, which involves not hanging out in the mall but foraging for food—the nutritious kind, not lichens.

Rudolf the Red-Eyed Reindeer

Like most wild herbivores, reindeer, which live in the Arctic, subarctic, and mountainous regions, have strong constitutions that are not just useful for pulling sleighs filled with toys. They have the ability to eat a variety of hallucinogenic plants and fungi without getting sick. Some of the mushrooms they eat are toxic to humans (unlike psilocybins, which have been popular with people) but not poisonous to the hardy reindeer. However, the use of psychoactive shrooms among reindeer is not without danger. The tripping beasts may wander away from their calves, for example, putting their offspring at risk of being devoured by wolves. (There are no calf-care services in the wild.)

During the Siberian summer, the reindeer feed on a variety of plants, but their favorite is the fly agaric, which grows in the birch forests. The animals embark on a hunt for these alluring red-capped mushrooms, which they ingest for their mind-blowing effects. Samorini reported in his field research that "the reindeer run around aimlessly, make strange noises, twitch their heads, and isolate themselves from the rest of the herd."

Humans, including native shamans who observed the caribou behaving strangely, decided to get in on the fun by eating the mushrooms themselves, causing them to cavort about like whacked-out wildebeests. For a more intense high, shamans would drink the urine of tripping reindeer. One assumes that, like beer served in England, reindeer urine is served warm rather than chilled.

Reindeer Games: Natural Highs

Reindeer are highly sociable, outgoing, and spirited animals. They gather in groups of hundreds and thousands so they can migrate from the tundra to the forests, where they can feast heartily. Some can even be domesticated and are said to be quite gentle, except during mating season, when males are likely to butt heads.

Gone Goats

Perhaps the most ardent drug users within the animal kingdom are goats, which partake of many forms of mind-altering drugs. Goats will devour psychedelic mushrooms (along with just about everything else left in their path). Goat herders are well aware of their charges' weakness for psilocybin, which is why they are careful not to leave home without a shepherd's crook. Apparently, the rambunctious rams have been known to attack anyone who comes between them and their shrooms. After consuming the fantasy-producing fungi, which they will eat exclusively if given the opportunity, the goats will become even more recalcitrant and dangerous, running around and shaking their heads crazily, like revelers at an *Animal House* frat party.

Silly Billy Goats: Natural Highs

Goats, like sheep, are social animals, and those who farm them or keep them at shelters say they can be quite friendly. The kids will jump playfully on their tolerant mothers' backs. They form strong bonds with people (unless they've been traumatized) and with other goats and sheep. A study published in *Animal Welfare* showed that they experience emotions, including boredom and happiness, in ways similar to humans, and that they pick up on emotional cues. So make sure you smile the next time you encounter a goat, especially one that seems wary.

Moths and Mollusks
Like to Get Lit

It is a well-known fact that moths are attracted to light, but I bet you didn't know that they also get drunk on the nectar of the datura flower, which is known for its hallucinogenic effects on humans. Botanists say the flower's power varies with the age of the plant.

Using their long proboscises, which act like straws, the moths suck in the flower's intoxicating nectar. Afterwards, they will fall to the ground, which puts them at risk of being swallowed by predators such as birds, bats, and rodents. It took hours of observation by researchers to conclude that the moths were, in fact, drunk from the nectar, probably because the datura plant blossoms open at night.

An article in the *Botanical Gazette* described the party this way: "They seem clumsy when they land on the flowers and often miss the target and fall onto the leaves or the soil. They right themselves slowly and awkwardly. When they take flight again, their movements are erratic, as if they were confused. But the moths seem to like this effect and return to suck more nectar from those flowers." The datura is apparently not just an open flower but an open bar, with the moths as ardent regulars.

Like the moth, slugs and snails also enjoy getting drunk. Many farmers and gardeners use alcohol to protect their crops by luring the mollusks with containers or saucers filled with beer or wine. The mollusks are enticed into these boozy traps, crawling from every direction to gather in their watery rave by the dozens, only to be swept up and unceremoniously disposed of.

Hedgehog Fun Managers

Clever farmers from Italy have used alcohol to attract hedgehogs into their gardens; they are welcome guests because they eat bugs that would otherwise devour cabbage and salad greens. Because these mammals are partial to alcohol, placing a bowl of watered-down wine (perhaps a nice Chianti) with a handful of tasty slugs in the middle of the garden creates a bucolic hedgehog buffet.

Hog Heaven

As cute as these spiny little critters can be, hedgehogs are not recommended as house pets, as they live only three years on average and do little more than curl up into a ball and sleep. They feast on a buffet of beetles, ants, termites, grasshoppers, moths, centipedes, and earthworms. Still, hedgehog owners say they can be handled by people (in time) and enjoy running in a wheel (no wire, solid surfaces only), playing with toilet paper tubes (if over three months of age), and playing with small, stuffed, child-safe toys. But like most exotic animals, they are better off (and happier) if left in the wild.

Monkey Business

Both capuchin monkeys in South America and lemurs in Madagascar have been known to get high off insects, including several species of millipedes that squirt out a poisonous compound when agitated. (Are you seeing a pattern yet with secreted toxins?) Lemurs and capuchins have discovered that they can ward off parasitic insects by covering themselves in the liquid, with the added bonus of getting a significant buzz. Consuming millipede poison, however, is risky business, as it is filled with cyanide, a compound deadly to pretty much every living thing. For many of these stoned simians, the mind-altering effect of the millipede juice is apparently worth the risk.

Monkey Around

Monkeys are almost synonymous with fun because they love to play. In the wild, where they should remain unless cared for by a zoologist, they climb trees, hang from vines, and swing to and from branches in search of bugs, fruits, and leaves. They are social and clean creatures that spend several hours a day removing parasites, dirt, or other material from one another's fur. They tend to sleep close to each other to form stronger bonds. As the infants grow, they play not only with monkeys but with other young animals. Young monkeys chase one another, wrestle, tumble, and play "king-of-the-castle," in which they take turns pushing each other off a high perch.

Gonzo Gorillas
and Bad-Ass Baboons

Primates will frequently forage for intoxicants in the wild when the desire strikes them. One of our closet animal relatives, the gorilla, has been seen digging roots of the iboga bush, which they are able to distinguish from other plants that grow copiously in the rainforest. The reason for the gorilla's fervent efforts to find and consume these bitter roots is that they produce intense psychoactive effects. Finding the nondescript rainforest bushes in the wild is no small feat, requiring sophisticated techniques that even the most seasoned botanist is unlikely to possess.

Similarly, the mandrill, which is closely related to the baboon and is found in rainforests in equatorial Africa, also digs the iboga bush. Shamans who live in these regions tell tales of iboga use among male mandrills. When a male engages in combat over a female, he will first find and dig up an iboga bush and eat its root before heading into battle. People in the region have taken to brewing these roots into an intoxicating beverage. (Do not tell Lance Armstrong or former Yankee A-Rod about the effects of the iboga.)

Scientists have reported that baboons will go to great lengths to find a rare, red, plum-like fruit belonging to the Cycadaceae family. The fruit, which is toxic to humans, is said to have an unpleasant odor that does not seem to put off the pleasure-seeking baboons, which strip the trees bare of this putrid crop to feast on. Afterwards, the baboons behave as though they are drunk, staggering like sailors on shore leave—oblivious to the dangers that surround them (such as hunters or dogs). Apparently, the feelings of euphoria that this fruit produces are enough to offset its foul taste.

Gorilla Games

The most important part of gorilla play is wrestling. Animals hug and hold onto each other, bite, hit, throw themselves onto their partner, and pull each other to the ground. This intense-sounding wrestling match is often accompanied by laughing, grunting, moaning, and panting noises. (Mandrills also enjoy play-fighting.) Young animals engage in such games more frequently than their elders, and adult females play least frequently, which will not surprise female readers. However, adult gorillas will join in on the fun if encouraged. (Yes, AARP members, our evolutionary cousins prove there is still fun after fifty.) Play is extremely important for young gorillas because it helps them familiarize themselves with others in order to be accepted as part of the group. Play helps them practice their communication skills and learn other patterns of behavior, not unlike play dates that help socialize human children.

Jaguar Junkies

Animal experts say that jaguars are the junkies of the jungle. These magnificent big cats will seek out the roots of the caapi plant found in South America and gnaw on them until they hallucinate. Caapi root contains a variety of powerful chemicals similar to those found in antidepressants that intensify the animal's senses. Some scientists believe that humans learned how to use the root by observing jaguars getting high. Shamans of the western Amazonian tribes have used the hallucinogenic plant in religious and healing ceremonies in an attempt to purge the body of parasites and aid the digestive tract.

Big Cats Naps

When it comes to play, big cats are similar to their domesticated cousins in that they stalk, hunt, sleep, and chase one another for amusement. When relaxed they can also be seen lying on their backs with their bellies toward the sky, but I would not recommend rubbing the tummy of a wild jaguar if you encounter one while on safari.

Wacky Wallabies

In the summer of 2009, Tasmanian farmers solved the mystery behind a bunch of crop circles, which, as it turned out, had nothing at all to do with aliens. The visitations and evisceration of crops were the result of stoned marsupials. Wallabies were caught eating opium poppies grown for medicinal purposes, not for heroin. They carved out crop circles as they hopped around all hopped up. Apparently, Tasmania produces half of the world's legally grown opium. One retired poppy farmer told the Australian Broadcasting Network that the animals "would just come and eat some poppies and they would go away. Then they'd come back again and do their circle work in the paddock."

Shadow Boxers

Wallabies, which are smaller members of the kangaroo clan, are found primarily in Australia and on nearby islands. Newborn Wallaby infants immediately crawl into their mothers' pouches, where they continue to develop after birth, usually for several months. Young wallabies and kangaroos are called joeys and are best known for their powerful legs, which allow them to jump high and travel great distances as a group. They also have the ability to play-box. When they are not hopping or punching, they show affection by licking and grooming one another.

Birds of a Feather Drink
(or Toke) Together

It might surprise some to learn that our feathered friends don't just fly high but like getting high. In the American West, for example, sapsuckers (a type of woodpecker) use their beaks to drill holes in trees in order to feast on sap. When exposed to a certain temperature, this sap will ferment, producing alcohol. Hummingbirds also get a buzz from the aforementioned datura flower.

The most well-known example of collective avian inebriation is found among robins during their annual migration in February to the warmer climes of California. One news account appeared in the small town of Pleasant Hill in the 1930s. After flying West, the flocks were seen perching on small ornamental trees known as California holly, which were flush with scarlet holly berries. The robins, and other birds, binged on the berries until they were drunk (I would say as a skunk, but skunks are teetotalers). This avian orgy continued unchecked for a full three weeks (apparently there is no law against winging under the influence), while birdwatchers observed helplessly as the disoriented robins fluttered about wildly—smashing into cars, windshields, and houses.

In his book *Intoxication*, Ronald Siegel notes that four or five holly berries would make a full meal for a single bird, but these ravenous robins will gorge on as many as thirty at a time, causing this scene: "They quickly work their way to the outermost branches, which begin to sag under their collective weight. As the branches wobble, so do the birds and they start falling. Four birds are staggering on the ground, unable to fly. . . . [Now] 18 birds on the ground. Several are still grasping berries in their beaks."

While robins tend to survive despite their bob, bob, bobbing, Samorini cites the studies of ornithologist David McKelvey that chronicled the decimation of the less fortunate pink pigeon, once native to the Mauritian Islands, that resulted from its desire for psychoactive plants and berries. According to McKelvey, the pigeons would feed on the berries and become incapacitated—incapable of doing anything but wandering around in a daze. When the

British introduced the mongoose to the islands, the pie-eyed pigeons turned into sitting ducks for these formidable carnivores, unable to fly out of harm's way.

Sparrows, on the other hand, are the stoners of the class, with a penchant for marijuana. Potheads will be pleased to learn that it gives the birds a much mellower and safer high. Sparrows have been known to swoop into storehouses to feed on hemp seeds, causing them to sing longer and with greater passion. In fact, some canary owners offer hemp seeds to their pets in order to make their songs sweeter, and parrot owners say it makes the birds more talkative. I would check with a vet before feeding hemp to your songbird, but now we know why the caged bird (sometimes) sings.

Love Birds

Many bird species are gregarious and form flocks for different reasons, but mostly for protection and survival. Flocks may be different sizes and can work well together in a group. Birds are caretakers not just of their young, but of each other, and can be seen preening their mates or other members of the flock. Robins will frequently sing in clear, lilting musical whistles. You can see robins scurrying across lawns or stalking earthworms in yards or parks. In winter they may seemingly disappear from sight but could still be around. Look for them in treetops and around fruiting trees and listen for their low notes. House sparrows are even more vocal than robins. They flutter down from eaves and fencerows to hop and peck at crumbs or birdseed.

Other birds, like parrots, toucans, and cockatiels, will play games such as fetch in a similar fashion to dogs. If you gently toss a small Koosh ball or a soft, lightweight toy in the direction of your parrot, it might very well run after the object and pick it up with its beak. They also enjoy swinging and climbing (ladders and bars of a cage, if domesticated, and branches and trees, if not). They are extremely emotional and will pine when their human companion is away, sometimes plucking their feathers until they are bald. They enjoy perching on a finger or shoulder, some can talk, and they are said to have the intelligence of an average three-year-old human.

Certain species of birds mate for life, including mute swans, whooping cranes, scarlet macaws, and bald eagles. Eagles have a spectacular courtship ritual in which they lock talons and then flip, spin, and twirl through the air in a maneuver called a cartwheel display. They break apart seemingly at the last moment, just before hitting the ground unharmed.

Beetle Juice

Ants, the Mensa members of the insect world, live in colonies and have the ability to work as a cooperative, industrious team. They have also developed a strange relationship with a species of beetle that they hospitably host in their nests. The Lomechusa beetle secretes an inebriating substance from its belly, which is so desired by ants that, should the colony be somehow disturbed by human or beast, they will forgo rescuing their precious larvae to protect the beetle. Clearly in need of Ants Anonymous, these creatures will drug themselves to the point where they will slack off from their vital work duties as protectors of the queen.

It Takes a Colony

Charles Darwin wrote, "In the long history of humankind [and animal kind, too] those who learned to collaborate and improvise most effectively have prevailed." Ants, which have been around for a hundred million years, are one of the finest examples of this evolutionary collaboration. As part of a matriarchal society, the female ants engage in a coordinated effort to ensure that all the queen's needs are met for the proper functioning of the entire colony. The males' role is to mate with the queen, after which they perish.

While some ants forage, others stay behind to tend the brood or to build, maintain, and defend the colony's living quarters. There are even mortician ants whose job it is to bury the dead. One might even say it is an anarchistic society because ants have no governing body to allocate and manage their activities. Their division of labor is not only successful but downright altruistic.

While ants are clearly pretty smart as a group, there's no recorded evidence of an ant library that documents the advantages of groupthink. One thing we humans do is think a lot (although you couldn't prove it during campaign season), and we have felt compelled to write down everything from our most mundane to our most profound thoughts, including what we think about pleasure. We'll take a whirlwind tour through some of that thinking in the next chapter.

4

The High Life

The Philosophy of Pleasure Seeking

There's an urban legend of unknown origin that's making the rounds on social media. Whether the story is true or not, the moral seems particularly apropos.

A professor stands before his philosophy class with several items on his desk. He picks up an empty mayonnaise jar and fills it with golf balls. He asks his students if the jar is full. They agree that it is. The professor then picks up a box of pebbles and pours them into the jar. He shakes the jar lightly. The pebbles roll into the open areas between the golf balls. He then asks the students again if the jar is full. They agree it is.

Next, the professor picks up a box of sand and pours it into the jar. The sand fills up the spaces around everything else. He asks once more if the jar is full. The students respond with a unanimous yes.

The professor then produces two bottles of beer from under the table and pours the entire contents into the jar, which gets absorbed by the sand. The students laugh.

"Now," says the professor as the laughter subsides, "I want you to recognize that this jar represents your life. The golf balls are the important things—your family, your health, your friends, and your passions. If everything else was lost and only these things remained, your life would still be full. The pebbles are the other things that matter, such as your work, your home, and your car. The sand is everything else—the small stuff.

"If you put the sand into the jar first," he continued, "there is no room for the pebbles or the golf balls. The same goes for life. If you spend all your time and energy on the small stuff, you will never have room for the things that are important to you. Pay attention to the things that are critical to your happiness. Spend time with your children. Spend time with your parents. Visit with grandparents. Take your spouse out to dinner. There will always be time to clean the house and mow the lawn. Take care of the golf balls first—the things that really matter. Set your priorities. The rest is just sand."

One of the students raised her hand and inquired what the beer represented. The professor smiled and said, "I'm glad you asked. The beer just shows you that no matter how full your life may seem, there's always room for a couple of beers with a friend."

There are several grains of truth within this parable, the most important being to focus on what gives us the most pleasure in life—family, friends, health, and our favorite passions (with the caveat that, if you're an alcoholic, a couple of beers would never be enough, so stick with your favorite soft drink). It's that simple. The pursuit of pleasure and happiness is something the big hitters of philosophy as well as modern thought leaders have had a lot to say about.

Ancient Wisdom

Philosophers throughout the ages—from Socrates to Buddha to the authors of Judaism's Kabbalah—were more than willing to advise others on how to live a happy life. These are all complex traditions, and I obviously can't do justice to them in the short summaries that follow. My purpose here is to pull out some pertinent ideas in an attempt to deepen your understanding of the role of pleasure in our lives.

The Good Greek Life

Socrates believed that reason was a path to the good life. He also told his followers to look inward (i.e., do some soul searching) to find happiness. Socrates was so convinced about the power of introspection that he famously declared, "the unexamined life is not worth living."

As far as our desires are concerned, Socrates said mere mortals have the ability to achieve "a divine-like state of inner tranquility." He was among the first philosophers to argue that happiness is not divinely given but humanly possible if we make an effort. Keep in mind that the ancient Greeks believed that happiness was extremely rare and reserved only for those the gods favored.

Against this somewhat gloomy backdrop, the optimistic Socrates believed that people were capable of harmonizing or prioritizing their desires to achieve this divine-like tranquility. By being virtuous and just, he said, one could realize the true purpose of human existence, which would then lead to a happier life. Most of us, he believed, are filled with pride, conceit, and beliefs we cling to for a sense of identity and security. Socrates challenged people's preconceived notions, most of which he felt were based on faulty logic. And who among us wants to argue with Socrates?

Socrates's student Plato wrote a number of famous dialogues on the pursuit of pleasure and happiness using his teacher as the central character. Scholars continue to debate the relationship between Socrates's original teachings and Plato's own ideas, but the following are the two ancients' deepest thoughts about pleasure and happiness:

- All human beings naturally desire happiness.
- Happiness is obtainable and teachable through effort.
- Happiness does not depend on material things but on how we use material goods (wisely or unwisely).
- Happiness depends on learning to harmonize our desires. We do this by giving more weight to our desire for knowledge and virtue than to our desire for physical pleasures.
- Virtue and happiness are inextricably linked; it is impossible to have one without the other.
- The pleasures we get from pursuing virtue and knowledge are on a higher plane than the pleasures we get from satisfying our baser desires. Pleasure is not the goal of existence, but it is an integral part of being virtuous.

The Greek word *eros* stands for love, friendship, and passion—desires that make up some of the best things in life. It is the root of the word "erotic" and, as you might guess, also includes sexual passion. While *eros* can keep us longing and never completely satisfied, Socrates said that we can either control it or let it take the wheel by letting our sexual desires overtake our reason. Jealousy, crimes of passion, and unrequited love are all examples of *eros* gone wild.

In Plato's *The Republic*, Socrates continues his discourse on the relationship between pleasure and virtue (morality). An immoral life, he says, is filled with guilt, stress, and anxiety—emotions that can lead us to escape through alcohol and other mood altering drugs. When you live a moral life, the philosopher says, you have peace of mind, but happiness also comes from the joy of knowledge, which involves exploring the higher realms of truth. Wisdom, he believed, can be far more rewarding than the pursuit of physical pleasure.

Socrates also theorized that nearly all pleasure is relative and that gratification can come from the absence of
pain. Let's say you are sick and suddenly get better; you
might consider your new condition to be pleasurable,
when it is simply a relief from illness. Of course, once you
get used to being well, it's no longer pleasurable. Likewise,
someone who gets a job after a long period of unemployment might find working pleasurable, while another person
who has the same job will find work a chore. Getting high
on drugs, which gives us satisfaction in the short term, will
eventually lead to pain if we abuse them, especially if we
become addicted. Perhaps it was Socrates who first coined
the phrase "it's all relative."

A century after Socrates and Plato, another Greek philosopher named Epicurus would expand on the argument
about positive and negative pleasures. Positive pleasure, he
submitted, is nothing more than the removal of pain. If you
are thirsty, you can drink a glass of water to get some relief.
Negative pleasure is that state of harmony where you no
longer feel any pain and therefore don't require a positive
pleasure (like a cool beverage) to get rid of the pain.

He maintained that positive pleasure always falls somewhere on a scale of good to great. This kind of pleasure can
also be frustrating, because there will always be a contrast
between the state you are now in and a "higher" state that
would make your current experience appear less desirable. If
you get more pleasure from sex than from eating, for example, eating won't seem as pleasurable (unless you're eating
during sex, I suppose). Epicurus concluded that the true
state of happiness is the state of negative pleasure, an oxymoron that is basically the absence of unfulfilled desires.
(This idea is similar to the Buddhist concept of achieving
Nirvana through the removal of desire. More about that
later.)

Plato had a renowned pupil, Aristotle, who proposed that pleasure is made up of *energeia,* which includes many activities such as music, art, and thinking, all of which help us lead fulfilling lives. He said the amount of pleasure we experience depends on how ardently we pursue certain activities. For example, as a beginning violinist gets better, the satisfaction she gets from playing music will also increase. Like his fellow philosophers, Aristotle believed some pleasures are greater than others. He ranked them as follows:

1. thinking
2. sight
3. hearing and smell
4. taste

Aristotle also argued that animals experience pleasures that are appropriate for their species; that is, a bear's pleasure is different from a dog's. Similarly, there are certain pleasures, such as the ones listed above, that are mainly for humans: thinking (contemplation), hearing (music), sight (art), smell (flowers/nature—although one could argue that animals enjoy this as well), taste (food—again, does anybody enjoy their food more than a dog?). We humans, on the other hand, can apply these ancient musings to our modern-day Pleasure Principles when deciding which activities we would like to pursue.

Epicurean Hedonism
If a little is not enough for you, nothing is.
—Epicurus

An article published in the *Journal of Happiness Studies* examines Epicurus's guide to the good life, which embraced the idea of hedonism—but not in the modern sense of the word, which is the belief that pleasure or happiness is the most important goal in life. Although Epicurus was a hedonist, he did not condone excessive pleasure-seeking. What Epicurus espoused was something more subtle; he did not believe that the road to happiness was paved with luxury or material wealth. What he emphasized was the idea that being "untroubled" was far superior to the pursuit of pleasure. His view was that pleasure and pain are so important to human existence that all our actions are governed either by seeking pleasure or avoiding pain (physical or psychological). Like Plato, Epicurus also saw the absence of pain as a pleasure in itself. He believed that true satisfaction could only be achieved when the body and mind are at peace.

So how did Epicurus suggest people achieve peace in both mind and body? To keep the body content and the mind free from fears, he advocated the following four-part strategy.

1. Don't fear the gods (or fate or chance).

Surprisingly, Epicurus's approach to the gods fits into our modern, more secular society. Epicurus felt the gods were already in a state of bliss and therefore disinterested in human activities. This being the case, humans had nothing to fear from the gods but should also expect nothing from them in return. It is up to each of us, he said, to create order in our lives, because the gods do not control us. In other words, we are responsible for our own lives and must manage our problems as they arise rather than leaving them in the hands of God or fate.

2. Don't worry about death.

Easier said than done, I know, but Epicurus had a (ahem) philosophical approach to death. He saw it as the end of our sensual (as in senses) experience and as a transition that should not concern us. While we are alive, death is not important, as it does not yet exist. Of course, we could get hit by a bus tomorrow, but until and unless that occurs, why worry about it? (It's a bit like being a teenager again—feeling invulnerable and invincible to harm.) Likewise, Epicurus argued, when we're dead, we no longer experience anything (including pain and suffering), so why not accept it and get on with your life (or death, as the case may be)? As you might have gathered by now, Epicurus did not believe in the afterlife or the soul's immortality.

3. What is good is easy to get.

Epicurus makes an important distinction between necessary and natural things, including our basic needs such as food and shelter. Unnecessary and unnatural things include fame, excessive wealth, or awards. (Listen up, Oscar winners!)

Even within the natural category, Epicurus made a distinction between the necessary and the unnecessary. Rice, which is available to people in even the poorest nations, will satisfy our hunger just as well as lobster. But if you've tasted lobster and can't afford to buy it, this could be a recipe for future unhappiness. That said, Epicurus wasn't completely against the occasional indulgence. He thought people who enjoyed the simple pleasures would be even more delighted by extravagances than a bon vivant. In most cases, however, he favored moderation.

Ultimately, Epicurus thought it better to learn how to be satisfied with life's simple pleasures because they are much easier to attain and they are likely to last longer, since good fortune can be fleeting. The more you have (or want), the more you have to lose.

4. What is terrible is easy to endure.

According to Epicurus, even physical pain can be endured by using the mind. Focusing on pleasure, he said, including gratification we have experienced in the past and what we might experience in the future, can help distract us from our bodily aches. Today this technique is called creative or positive visualization.

The Laughing Buddha

Budai, or Pu-Tai, is nicknamed the Laughing Buddha in Chinese because he is almost always shown smiling or chuckling. Budai carries few possessions other than prayer beads and whatever he has in his cloth sack; he is poor but content. He is often shown entertaining or being followed by adoring children. This jolly deity is admired by Buddhists for his happiness and prosperity. According to folklore, rubbing his round belly brings wealth and good fortune. He is seen by some believers as the future Buddha, but he should not be confused with Siddhārtha Gautama, the prophet who is considered the founder of Buddhism.

Buddhists believe that all beings possess "Buddha nature" within them, which is to say that we are already enlightened, even if we've yet to realize it. During his life, Buddha experienced both intense pleasure and extreme deprivation, but he found that neither extreme leads to a true understanding. He practiced meditation under a bodhi tree, where he found enlightenment. After that, he began teaching the Four Noble Truths to others in order to help them achieve happiness and peace of mind. The Four Noble Truths according to Buddhism are:

1. Life involves *dukkha* (mental dysfunction or suffering).
2. *Dukkha* arises from craving.

3. *Dukkha* can be eliminated.

4. The way to the elimination of *dukkha* is the Eightfold Path.

The Eightfold Path is often divided into three categories: wisdom (right view/understanding, right intention), ethical conduct (right speech, right action, right livelihood), and mental cultivation (right effort, right mindfulness, right concentration).

When we crave things, whether material goods or getting high, we are attempting to fill an inner void. Drugs and alcohol might provide brief satisfaction, but it never lasts, and, for some, it is never enough—so we crave more. There is a Sanskrit word for this paradox, *upadana,* which refers to a cycle of craving and grasping. As the Buddha's path of wisdom states: "The craving of one given to heedless living grows like a creeper. Like the monkey seeking roots in the forest, he leaps from life to life. . . . Whoever is overcome by the wretched and sticky craving, his sorrows grow like the grass after the rains." Or as the Dalai Lama recommends: "It is better to want what you have than to have what you want."

The *sutta* (a discourse of the Buddha) known as "The Arrow" further explores Buddhist attitudes toward pleasure and pain. When we encounter something that leads to pain (or even just dissatisfaction), we tend to produce thoughts that lead to more suffering, often increasing our pain. This leads us to indulge in blame, criticism, and complaining. It has been compared to being shot by an arrow and then shooting ourselves with another arrow. (The Western equivalent might be shooting oneself in the foot.) A wiser course of action, according to Buddhists, is to avoid the second arrow by allowing yourself to feel discomfort without reacting to it. This concept obviously requires practice and mental discipline, which are offered in the Eightfold Path and other Buddhist teachings.

Most of us know what it's like to experience something pleasurable that makes us want to return to the source of our enjoyment. (This becomes an endless compulsive cycle in the case of addiction.) Because all pleasure is temporary, this craving for whatever pleasure we seek can end up causing us pain if we overindulge. The best path to follow, especially if you have an addictive personality, Buddhists suggest, is to remain emotionally neutral. This is known as equanimity, which doesn't mean we cultivate a machine-like inability to feel. Rather, it's a way to break bad habits and patterns when it comes to thoughts and emotions that can cause us pain. It is only when we experience this freedom, Buddhists believe, that we become happier.

Finding the Truth Brought Peace
Best hobby is to practice Buddhism in everyday life.
I was depressed for two years and the only thing that got me out was wisdom and insight of Buddhism.
I was able to look inside me, understand myself better, understand others better, and understand how the world around me was operating. No situation around me changed, but mere understanding the truth of things gave me incomparable peace and serenity. Nothing can give more happiness in life than being close to TRUTH.

—Anonymous

Hindu Happiness
It's not surprising that the religion responsible for the *Kama Sutra*, a manual for erotic and other human pleasures,

would thoroughly embrace the pursuit of sensuality and desire. Hindus believe that pleasure is just one of four essential goals in life. They are:

1. *Dharma*: fulfilling one's purpose.

2. *Artha*: wealth, career, financial security, and economic prosperity. The proper pursuit of *artha* is an important aim of human life in Hinduism.

3. *Kama*: desire, sexuality, enjoyment. Although *kama* primarily refers to romantic love and sexual pleasure, it also encompasses desire in general. Some schools of Hinduism teach that *kama* is a worthy pursuit when it's done with special disciplines that result in higher insight into its source.

4. *Moksha*: enlightenment. *Moksha* involves freedom and self-knowledge.

The Sanskrit word *dharma* means many things, including one's destiny or purpose. But Hindus also believe that we are born indebted to the gods and various humans and that we must repay karmic debts during our lifetime. These debts include the blessings from the gods, which are repaid through rituals and offerings. Parents and teachers are repaid by their children and by passing along knowledge; guests are repaid by being treated hospitably; humans are repaid through respect; and all other living beings are repaid through goodwill, food, or assistance, if needed. *Dharma* also means righteousness, or living morally and ethically at all times, which most religions would also condone.

Kabbalah

Kabbalah, which means "to receive and to accept," is a Jewish philosophy dating back to the sixteenth century and popularized in eighteenth-century Hassidic practices. It embraces many of the Pleasure Principles, including revitalizing the mind, body, and spirit. Kabbalah was founded on the belief that we are here to fulfill a mission to improve ourselves and that we all possess the knowledge and the ability to achieve emotional, spiritual, and physical well-being. It is based on the idea that humans possess both an animal (physical) and a spiritual soul that will help guide us toward living a healthier, happier life. A central tenet of Kabbalah is the Tree of Life, which contains the ten levels of human existence:

1. *Keter (Crown):* Our highest self. This is the level to which we should all aspire. Some Kabbalists call *keter* our guardian angel or spiritual guide because it never gives up on us and is always trying to lead us toward our true purpose in life. When we are not living up to our highest self or purpose we are likely following our animalistic soul, which desires physical satisfaction (e.g., food, sex, or material goods), instead of following our spiritual soul. Kabbalists believe that we can stop our destructive habits and discover who we were meant to be. This return to the right path is called *teshuva* in Hebrew.

2. *Hokhma (Wisdom):* Our spirituality and intuition. In this level we explore our own spirituality by making space and time for it in our lives.

3. *Binah (Understanding):* Our rational and intellectual selves. *Binah* is a basic human need to acquire knowledge, be it learning a new skill, another language, or how to play an instrument, or trying new recipes. This channel must be kept open so we can grow.

4. *Chesed (Kindness):* Our loving, generous, and charitable spirit. Things you can do to reach this level include being grateful for the blessings in your life and being generous and charitable to others.

5. *Gevura (Judgment)*: Our ability to be disciplined, set boundaries, and manage time and money.

6. *Tiferet (Beauty and Peace)*: *Tiferet* involves guarding and maintaining our inner peace. People perceive truth and reality in different ways, but we all have the power to create our happiness and to live in harmony, according to Kabbalah. To achieve *tiferet* requires balance, spirituality, integration, beauty, and compassion.

7. *Netzah (Victory and Endurance)*: *Netzah* involves the creativity in our work and everyday life. Most of us have to engage in mundane tasks, such as housecleaning, shopping, laundry, and other chores. But the Kabbalah says there is a creative spark within all of us if we choose to release it.

8. *Hod (Glory)*: Our living environment and domestic spirit. The clothes we wear and how we choose to decorate our home are just two layers of our true self. The Kabbalah advises us to pay attention to our environment by surrounding ourselves with things that inspire us and make us feel good. When sitting down to a meal, for example, using attractive table settings, such as flowers and good silverware, will help create a more pleasurable and relaxing experience.

9. *Yesod (Foundation)*: Our relationships, sexuality, and communication. According to the Zohar, a two-thousand-year-old spiritual text used by Kabbalists to explain the secrets of the Torah, the universe, and everyday life: "If a person smiles, Heaven smiles at him; if he is sad and depressed, Heaven judges him with strictness." This is a simple yet profound example of how to add joy to your life and others' lives.

10. *Malchut (Kingship)*: Physical body and health. *Malchut* receives its energy from all of the above and is about nourishing our body and health. When we fall short in any of the higher levels, it has an impact on our physical well-being.

According to the Kabbalah, there are three "garments" of the soul: action, speech, and thought. We have the ability to control them all. With every act we perform, every word we speak, and every thought that enters our mind, we release energy—be it positive or negative. When we create positive energy, we open ourselves up to the blessings in our lives. Likewise, negative energy begets negativity, and if left unchecked, it will define who we are, which translates into how others see us.

Modern Thinkers, Spiritual Leaders, and Happiness Gurus

While we can look to philosophers and prophets to help us find the path to guilt-free pleasures, we can also pay attention to what some of the modern religious and secular thought leaders have to say about getting on board a higher plane to the high life.

In a recent interview with the Argentine publication *Viva*, Pope Francis offered advice for being a happier person, based on his own life experiences. He encouraged people to be more positive and generous, to turn off the TV and find healthier forms of leisure, and, refreshingly, to stop trying to convert people to your own particular beliefs. The following are his top ten tips for a happier life.

1. *"Live and let live."* Pope Francis gave the following advice, which comes from an Italian cliché meaning, "Move forward and let others do the same": "Everyone should be guided by this principle," he said. This is also one of the slogans that people in both AA and Al-Anon use to keep themselves grounded in their program of recovery.

2. *"Be giving of yourself to others."* People need to be open and generous toward others, he said, because "if you withdraw into yourself, you run the risk of becoming egocentric. And stagnant water becomes putrid."

3. *"Proceed calmly" in life.* The pope, a former high school literature teacher, used an example from an Argentine novel by Ricardo Guiraldes, in which the protagonist, rancher Don Segundo Sombra, looks back on how he lived his life. In the story Don Sombra proposes new ethical examples to a youth the author considered disoriented and restless, including this advice.

4. *A healthy sense of leisure.* The pope said, "Consumerism has brought us anxiety," and told parents to set aside time to play with their children and to turn off the TV when they sit down to eat.

5. *Sundays should be holidays.* Workers should have Sundays off because "Sunday is for family," he said.

6. *Find innovative ways to create dignified jobs for young people.* "We need to be creative with young people. If they have no opportunities they will get into drugs" and be more vulnerable to suicide, he said.

7. *Respect and take care of nature.* Environmental degradation "is one of the biggest challenges we have," he said. "I think a question that we're not asking ourselves is: 'Isn't humanity committing suicide with this indiscriminate and tyrannical use of nature?'"

8. *Stop being negative.* "Needing to talk badly about others indicates low self-esteem. That means, 'I feel so low that instead of picking myself up I have to cut others down,'" the pope said. "Letting go of negative things quickly is healthy."

9. *Don't proselytize; respect others' beliefs.* "We can inspire others through witness so that one grows together in communicating. But the worst thing of all is religious proselytism, which paralyses. . . . The church grows by attraction, not proselytizing," the pope said.

10. *Work for peace.* "We are living in a time of many wars," he said, and "the call for peace must be shouted. Peace

sometimes gives the impression of being quiet, but it is never quiet, peace is always proactive" and dynamic.

The Dalai Lama, another beloved spiritual leader, who travels the world teaching his Tibetan brand of Buddhism, had this to say about achieving pleasure and happiness:

> We all want happiness, not suffering, and as a consequence we have to see if the mind can be transformed. . . . There's no reason to feel low or demoralized; much better to be confident and optimistic. . . . I believe compassion to be one of the few things we can practice that will bring immediate and long-term happiness to our lives. I'm not talking about the short-term gratification of pleasures like sex, drugs or gambling (although I'm not knocking them), but something that will bring true and lasting happiness. The kind that sticks.

So what defines someone as an optimist or a pessimist other than the glass-half-full-or-empty test? Scientific studies have shown that those who have a Pollyanna personality believe that negative events are temporary and limited in scope, rather than pervading every aspect of a person's life, and that most problems are manageable and not out of one's control.

Wherever you fall on the scale, professor of positivity Martin Seligman, director of the Positive Psychology Center at the University of Pennsylvania, says that optimism is a *learned* skill and that people can train themselves to be happier by changing the way they think and perceive the world. He cites recent studies that have shown how optimistic people are happier, have more social support, and feel less stressed and less depressed. Like the Dalai Lama, Seligman says optimists react to problems with a sense of confidence rather than with a sense of defeat (e.g., "This will work out" versus "Everything bad always happens to me.")

Eckhart Tolle, a spiritual teacher and best-selling author of *The Power of Now* and *A New Earth*, takes a slightly different view, although he also believes that our thoughts are directly connected to our happiness. He is guided by the precepts that involve living in the moment and clearing one's mind of all thoughts, both positive and negative, to maintain emotional "neutrality." He says living in the moment has given him the gift of true peace and contentment.

"Pleasure is always derived from something outside you, whereas joy arises from within," Tolle explains. "The primary cause of unhappiness is never the situation but the thought about it. Be aware of the thoughts you are thinking. Separate them from the situation, which is always neutral. It is as it is."

He also advises people who are frequently caught in a maelstrom of negative thoughts and worries to, literally, stop and smell the flowers: "Look at a tree, a flower, a plant," he suggests. "Let your awareness rest upon it. How still they are, how deeply rooted in Being. Allow nature to teach you stillness."

Another purveyor of positivity is Gretchen Rubin, the Yale-trained lawyer and author of the wildly popular *The Happiness Project: Or, Why I Spent a Year Trying to Sing in the Morning, Clean My Closets, Fight Right, Read Aristotle, and Generally Have More Fun*. (Apparently Rubin sought the wisdom of Greek philosophers.) Like Tolle and other satisfaction seekers, Rubin says that simple pleasures give us the greatest contentment and that we must learn to "appreciate our ordinary day." Before you embark on your journey to find happiness, Rubin says you should ask yourself:

- What makes you feel good? What gives you joy, energy, fun?

- What makes you feel bad? What brings you anger, guilt, boredom, dread?
- What makes you feel right? What values do you want your life to reflect?
- How can you build an atmosphere of growth—where you learn, explore, build, teach, help?

Self-reflective questions like these can help us pinpoint the areas in our lives that might be causing us pain, frustration, or anxiety, and help us achieve that feeling of bliss that we all crave.

Offering more insight into living what she calls a "wholehearted life" is psychologist and author Brené Brown, whose TED Talks have drawn more than fifteen million views online. Her lectures and best-selling books on vulnerability, courage, worthiness, and shame have one common denominator, which is learning how to love oneself. It might sound trite at first, but it is the basic foundation on which we build our self-esteem and confidence—two critical elements to happiness.

Brown says that people who live wholeheartedly will sometimes feel exhausted and overwhelmed, but they can become deliberate in their thoughts and behaviors through prayer, meditation, or simply seeing their intentions. The greatest gift, she says, is being able to recognize shame when it's happening. (And as we know, shame and pain can cause us to self-medicate.) She suggests sharing your "shame story" with someone who has earned the right to hear it (i.e., someone you can trust) and someone you can count on to respond with compassion. She says this is all we need to cultivate courage, compassion, and connection.

Many modern thinkers reflect on human suffering and the craving for pleasure and escape. One of the most prominent gurus today is Deepak Chopra, the Indian American physician who practices holistic health and meditation as a means for finding peace and happiness. "Life can never be total pleasure," Chopra says. "Pain is always mixed in, and if you want to solve the negative aspects of life—everything that is shoved away to fester in the darkness of the shadow—you must go beyond pleasure."

The Chopra Addiction and Wellness Center, based in Vancouver, British Columbia, incorporates his theories on the healing power of meditation and reflection. The Center's credo is that, no matter what form they take, all addictions are rooted in the desire to satisfy our need for security, comfort, and love.

Whatever philosophy or spiritual path you decide to follow, most spiritual seekers seem to agree that we all have the ability to feel joy, which requires a harmony of mind, body, and spirit. The life worth living involves fun, love, laughter, companionship, compassion, and movement, as well as stillness and reflection. Philosophically speaking, our sadness and pain stem from the notion that nothing can fully satisfy our desires, much like that mythical professor's jar, which is filled with all the pleasures in life we need to be happy, and yet we continue to want more.

If you are using drugs or alcohol for pleasure, you are on a crash course to pain and suffering. You will never find happiness in a bottle, line, or bowl, although it might make you feel better temporarily. If it's real, long-lasting happiness you desire (and who doesn't?), the ideas explored in this chapter can give you food for positive thought and prepare for the next main course in part 2—the pursuit of the six Pleasure Principles.

Guilt-Free Highs

*Follow your bliss and the universe will open doors
where there were only walls.*

—Joseph Campbell,
American writer, mythologist, lecturer

Now that you understand that the search for pleasure and
escape is a universal drive, some of you might think that
mood-altering chemicals are to happiness what the four
major food groups are to nutrition—that they're essential
for avoiding a life of mirthless deprivation. But the truth,
I'm pleased to report, is that natural highs are not only
abundantly available but better, stronger, cheaper, and
longer lasting than the ones we get from alcohol or drugs.
The nearly five hundred people surveyed or interviewed for
this book spoke lovingly about some of their favorite natural highs, which included socializing and celebrating with
friends and family, laughing, having sex, engaging in some
kind of exercise or sport, dancing, singing, volunteering, flying a plane, and, for one enthusiast, swinging on a trapeze.

These guilt-free highs are all part of the six Pleasure
Principles explored in this section: Move, Restore, Connect, Create, Celebrate, and Give. There are more than six,
of course, but let's call this a short list for finding bliss.
Whether it's thrill-seeking pleasures or a mellower buzz you
seek, there are myriad ways to get the emotional, physical,
and spiritual satisfaction—experiencing your whole self as
mind, body, and spirit—without the use of alcohol or other
drugs. In a national, unscientific survey of 432 men and
women, ages twenty-five to sixty-four, which was commis-
sioned from Survata Inc. for this book, 72 respondents said
laughter gave them the most pleasure, followed by sex (54),
with socializing coming in third (47). It should be noted
that creative pursuits such as music, art, writing, and so

forth, were in a near dead-heat for third place with 45 votes. Not only do these Pleasure Principles produce the same mood-elevating effects as drugs, many have been scientifically shown to reduce depression and stress. One thing we all share is pain, which everyone experiences at some point in his or her life. Loved ones get sick, die, or desert us. We sometimes get ill or injured. Jobs are lost, unrewarding, or seemingly impossible to get.

But keep in mind not all pain or stress is a bad thing to be medicated away. Pain can be a red flag that prompts us to see a doctor to treat a potentially serious health issue. Similarly, some stress allows us to discover ways to overcome the inevitable obstacles we face; it gives us the opportunity to dig deep and cultivate growth, self-efficacy, and self-esteem. Chronic stress (the kind that is ongoing), on the other hand, can weaken our immune system and make us more susceptible to illnesses, including ulcers, asthma, diabetes, and heart disease. It also increases our desire to self-medicate.

Unlike Carrie Nation, who preached the evils of alcohol, I believe that unless you're an alcoholic or addict, a few glasses of wine or beer or a cocktail or two at the end of the day or at a special event can enhance your enjoyment of a meal or the event. I'm offering the following Pleasure Principles, which have been proven to reduce the bad stress in your life, increase your resilience (especially if you are currently using or in recovery), and help you resist the siren call of artificial chemical boosts as your principal source of pleasure and escape. Many of the people who contributed their stories chose to remain anonymous, but they are real people whose testimonials are meant to inspire you to live the authentic high life.

Pleasure Principle #1

Move

Inhabiting the Body
through Physical Activity

*Competition to be the best individually and as a team,
that's what gives me my high—I know that if I work
really hard, and I can refine some things in my game,
then I can shoot to try and be the best.*

—Tim Howard, goalkeeper,
US National Soccer Team

You already know that exercise is good for your heart and your health, but did you know that it's also good for your head and your spirit? Countless studies have conclusively shown that people who boost their heart rates through exercise also lower their risk of depression and anxiety. Why does exercise keep us so happy and calm? One reason is the increased blood flow releases feel-good neurotransmitters, including endorphins, or "endogenous morphine" (you read that correctly), the brain's natural opioids that produce feelings of euphoria and well-being. Simply put—the more you exercise, the better and more rewarding the high.

"If you talk to people after an intense workout they will describe a feeling of relaxation, a sense of well-being, and ability to focus better," says Matt Bellace, a neuropsychologist from Princeton, New Jersey, and author of *A Better High*. "Endorphins give you the same feeling you get when you are high—the difference is that exercise will improve your memory and it's safer, especially for the adolescent brain."

The good news for exercise haters is that you don't have to run a marathon (or even break a sweat) to get a brain buzz (although it's better if you do break a sweat). Research has shown that as little as twenty minutes of walking can do the trick. One Norwegian survey published in 2013 found that those who engaged in any kind of exercise, even a small amount, reported improved mental health compared with people who—despite the alluring Scandinavian mountains and fjords—chose a sedentary lifestyle. According to another recent study from the American College of Sports Medicine (ACSM), moderately intense aerobic exercise immediately improves your mood, and that lift in spirit can last for up to twelve hours. The ACSM also discovered that six weeks of bicycle riding or weight training helped ease symptoms in women who were diagnosed with anxiety disorder. Weight training was especially effective for reducing feelings of irritability. In fact, some neurologists say that exercise can work better than antidepressants, and without the negative side effects, which might include drowsiness, blurred vision, nausea, impotence, and weight gain. Not only does moving your body help relieve anxiety, it also enhances concentration, learning, and memory—you might call these positive side effects.

While exercise is one of the best ways to get a natural high, I understand there are many out there who, unlike that old Bruce Springsteen song, are definitely not born to run. But if you can muster up the inspiration to get moving, I guarantee that you'll feel better about yourself (and your body). If the only exercise you currently do is with your thumbs on your smartphone, or doing fork-lifts of food into your mouth, and you haven't exercised in a long time (or ever), consult a doctor before starting. The same goes for people who don't exercise because of pain or injuries. As it turns out, the longer we continue to work out, the greater our tolerance for discomfort. New findings suggest that as muscles begin to ache during an extended workout, those natural opiates, such as endorphins and other substances, can help ease our pain. In other words, exercise can be a natural alternative to potentially addictive painkillers. This effect usually begins during the workout and lasts for approximately twenty or thirty minutes afterwards. That said, you should consult with a doctor before beginning any exercise regimen, especially if you have a preexisting injury or condition.

For those who suffer from arthritis, tendinitis, back pain, or other such conditions, exercise can be difficult but not impossible. A good physical therapist can help you find stretches that will help relieve your pain and make you stronger. Moving arthritic joints actually helps improve your range of motion while strengthening the muscles around the joint. Similarly, stretching back muscles will also help promote healing. Aqua therapy (water therapy), water aerobics classes, and swimming in general can offer a low-impact, painless way to reduce pain, get you moving, and improve your mood. Whatever your disability or physical challenge, don't give up—get up!

In the rest of this chapter, we'll take a look at some common (and not so common) ways people everywhere have found to move their bodies and raise their spirits. Pick and choose to suit your interests, physical capacity, and lifestyle.

Walk It Off

Whether it's around the park, around the block, or around the mall, whenever you are feeling tense or anxious—walk it off! It sometimes helps to have a walking buddy, so grab a friend, a group of friends, or your partner and start a regular walking group. Making your daily constitutionals a group activity turns exercise into a social activity, which combines two Pleasure Principles, especially if you think going for a stroll is a bore or a chore. Jane Brody, the *New York Times* personal health columnist, now seventy, wrote the following about her cherished daily walks with friends:

> Shortly after 6 the other morning, a stunning full moon hugging the horizon enhanced our walk around our local park, and I remarked, "Look what the stay-a-beds are missing." . . . Note that I said "[our]." Two to five of us walk for an hour every morning. We chat about our days, share our thoughts and problems, seek and offer advice, bolster sagging spirits, provide logistical support, alert one another to coming cultural events, discuss the news, books, articles and what-have-you. No matter how awful I may feel when I get up in the morning, I always feel better after that walk.

Newbies can improve their endurance by walking for ten seconds at a faster clip and then letting their body recover before speeding up again. Depending on your time and fitness level, you can increase your stamina by walking a little bit farther every day, week, or month. If you want to get your heart pumping, try speed walking, which is quickening your pace while swinging your bent arms in an exaggerated motion back and forth. It might feel (and look) a bit awkward at first, but who cares—it's good for your physical and mental health.

You can incorporate walking into almost any activity, so saying you don't have the time is no excuse. Fast walk on your way to the bus stop, while pushing a baby stroller (get one that is especially made for running and join a group of other parents and tots who are hot to trot). Add some ankle weights while you're walking, and you've upped the ante (you can hide them under your pant legs). Strap on a pedometer that counts every step you take, and watch the numbers tick up along with your ticker. Competitive types can make a contest out of seeing who got the highest number in a day. The winner can take the others out for lunch (no fast food—just fast walking) or coffee.

If you want to take it up a notch while doing errands, park your car in the spot that is the farthest away from your destination, and hoof it. I always laugh when I see people looking for the closest parking space to the entrance of the gym where they are about to work out on a treadmill or StairMaster. Speaking of, take the stairs instead of the elevator. If you're on the escalator, politely pass the riders and walk up the fast lane on the left. Soccer moms and dads can take a few spins around the periphery of the field during their children's sports games instead of dipping into the snack bag. Your kids shouldn't be the only ones getting exercise.

Be a Team Player

If you are feeling lonely and sad, nothing is more uplifting than a game of soccer, softball, volleyball, touch football, kickball, or basketball. You will spend time with other active types and get that feeling of camaraderie and morale boost that comes with assisting and cheering on a fellow player. Unfortunately, women are still not as likely to get involved in team sports as men, although this is rapidly changing with the popularity of children's soccer and Little League, which get young girls leaning in early in the game. And men, especially as they get older, are overwhelmingly more likely to be spectators rather than players, preferring the stadium or sports bar to being on the field. That said, if you need a little motivation, co-ed teams are a great way to meet potential dates, and couples (even old marrieds) can feel they are playing on the same team again after a good game of doubles.

The Runner's High

Nearly everyone has heard about the runner's high—the endorphin rush that comes from going for a heart-pumping, endurance run. In fact, avid runners swear that their sweat-soaked exercise produces the same feeling as mood-altering drugs. Some say they feel relaxed or at peace after running, while others—mostly those who run long-distance or race in marathons—say they feel euphoric. Medical technology now confirms these anecdotal reports of the runner's high. Researchers in Germany, using advances in neuroscience, reported in the journal *Cerebral Cortex* that running does, unquestionably, release a flood of endorphins in the brain. The endorphins are associated with mood changes, and the more endorphins a runner pumps out, the greater the effect.

One woman reported having such volatile emotions after completing a marathon that she broke into tears at the sight of a puppy. Others experience this hormonal high when pushing themselves to the point of exhaustion, which usually happens during sprints or interval training lasting up to two minutes. This triggers the production of lactic acid, which is known as anaerobic exercise and is said to improve heart strength and endurance.

I realize that running is not for everyone (I prefer spinning for my cardio fix), and it can be hard on the joints, especially as we age, although new research suggests a little pounding on the joints helps keep them stronger. And some people who have not been training or who push themselves too hard can also feel nauseated after a run—but not nearly as often as when overindulging in alcohol and other drugs. And there's no hangover after a good run. For athletes and nonathletes alike, these findings offer hope for those who do not enjoy exercise but might want to do it anyway—just for the hormonal buzz. These exercisers might learn techniques to elicit a feeling that makes working out positively addictive. As with anything that alters our mood, running can indeed become compulsive to the point of being addictive in an unhealthy way. If it becomes an obsession to the point of affecting your health and interfering with other parts of your life, but you keep doing it anyway, then it's time to get help to moderate your activities—or find another way to exercise that is part of a balanced life.

**Tiffany, Age Thirty-Five,
Public Relations Professional from Illinois**
I finally quit my coke habit when I was in my twenties through exercise. I joined a gym where I worked with a trainer, who was also a former coke addict. I told her my situation, and it was our mission to get me off the drug. I worked out like crazy doing weight lifting and cardio. Exercise gave me the same feeling I got when I was high, so I eventually weaned myself off cocaine. I haven't touched the stuff in a decade. The only drug I

do now is pot, which I smoke socially, and drink, which I also do socially. I can have pot and alcohol in the house, but it never occurs to me to use either unless I have a friend over who wants to indulge.

Jump for Joy

Jumping rope is one of the easiest and cheapest ways to get a good cardio workout without joining a gym or leaving your home. Make sure your downstairs neighbors are away if you live in an apartment. Also, buy a pair of good athletic shoes (preferably cross trainers) because jumping can put a lot of stress on your calves, ankles, and legs. Women may need a supportive sports bra.

Jump for a full three minutes with a one-minute break after each round. Work up to jumping three times a day, five days a week, if possible. Give yourself at least two weeks to get it right, and try not to take extra jumps in between swings. "Jump light, imagining that hot coals are under each foot," legendary boxer Sugar Ray Leonard told AARP. Use a heavier jump rope with a sturdy rubber grip. Jumping with lighter rope is actually more difficult, especially for beginners. Former professional boxer Yuri Foreman recommends an Altus 9-foot or the Body Solid Speed Jump Rope, which you can order online or at a sporting goods store.

You'll need a four-by-six-foot area and at least ten inches of space above your head. The exercise surface you jump on is very important. Do not attempt to jump on carpet, grass, concrete, or asphalt. While carpet reduces impact, it can also take hold of your shoes, which puts you at risk of twisting an ankle or knee. Your best bet is a wood floor or an impact mat made for exercise available at a sporting goods store or online.

The Need for Speed

*For me, personally, skiing holds everything. I used to race cars,
but skiing is a step beyond that. It removes the machinery
and puts you one step closer to the elements.
And it's a complete physical expression of freedom.*

—Robert Redford, actor,
founder of the Sundance Film Festival

Because exercise should be fun, the best way to ensure that you stick with any program is to find an activity that you enjoy doing and might become passionate about. Many people like the adrenaline rush that comes with adventure sports. Thrill seekers are usually born not made, but if you've always wanted to ski, scuba dive, board (skate or snow), blade, or rock climb, why not give it a try? Whether it's scaling mountains or exploring the depths of the ocean, it's never too late to start, as long as you take the proper precautions, which includes taking lessons, having the right gear from head to toe, and having an experienced guide to show you the ropes or slopes, depending on the sport.

Catch a High Wave

In addition to being a neuropsychologist, Matt Bellace is also a comedian; he works in two highly stressful professions. His exercise of choice is riding the waves. "I used to be a runner, but now surfing is my favorite natural high," he says. "It helps me manage my anxiety, which I have a lot of. There's kind of a meditative quality about surfing. I'm out there on my own, just me and my breath, and when I catch a wave there's this exhilaration that makes me shout with excitement. I feel good for about a week afterwards and walk around beaming. Part of the high is being in nature and part is the energy you exert from paddling. It's a multiple high! It's empowering to feel that surge of emotion when riding the waves. When you use drugs, they knock you out. A wave might knock you down, but natural highs like surfing just make you feel happier and healthier."

Kathy Gruver, Author of *Conquer Your Stress with Mind/Body Techniques*

I started doing the trapeze a little over a year ago, and nothing beats the feeling of flying through the air and connecting to do a catch. I like doing thrilling activities and the rush of being taken out of my comfort zone. Whether it's skydiving or ziplining, there's something so appealing about flying through the air in a safe environment. I like to encourage my clients to take healthy, smart risks by trying new things. Taking risks spills over into other parts of our lives as well. People who do things that make them uncomfortable become happier people. With every new thing we try the more confident and fulfilled we feel. You will feel like you have the courage to do anything.

It sounds weird, but I actually feel mentally clear when I do these types of activities. There is that initial feeling of stress, especially with something like skydiving, but then those fabulous hormones kick in, and I definitely feel high. It's the adrenaline rush, plus that sense of accomplishment that I did something so unique and cool. The first time my girlfriend and I went skydiving we were high the rest of the day. To me, the trapeze is a moving meditation of body, mind, and spirit coming together to do something really fun and adventurous.

Spin City

Unless you've been dosing for the last two decades, you've probably heard about spinning, which was invented by

South African Johnny Goldberg, better known as Johnny G. Johnny G moved to California, where he developed a special stationary bike with a weighted fly wheel that has become a mean, sweat-producing exercise machine. Unlike the recumbent bicycle, where riders can sit back, read, text, or watch TV, spinning is an all-in workout that simulates an outdoor ride with its snug seat and forward-leaning handle bars. You can adjust the tension on the wheel to increase the resistance when you want to feel as if you're riding uphill.

Place an instructor on a platform in front of a peloton of spinners, crank up your favorite playlist, and you've got yourself a forty-five-minute cardio party. Most gyms across the country have some form of spinning class (often called studio cycling), which have stood the test of time, unlike step aerobics, slides, trampolines, Tae Bo, and other fleeting exercise trends. Not only does spinning pump up your heart rate and burn up calories when the flywheel hits the imaginary road, it has become a form of therapy for enthusiasts, some of whom must reserve a bike twenty-four hours in advance in order to secure a spot. Although popular with Type A's, there is no competition involved other than beating your personal best, and you can design your own workout to make it age- and fitness-appropriate. If you are pregnant or have a preexisting condition, consult a doctor before going for a spin. The following are some things to keep in mind to get the most out of your ride:

Height matters. The biggest mistake spinners make is to setting the bike seat too low, which puts too much pressure on your knees. When pedaling, the leg should be bent about 25 degrees at the bottom of the rotation. Ask your instructor to help you adjust the bike for your height, and remember the settings for the next time you go to class.

Don't spin out of control. In the beginning Johnny G created the spinning bike, and it was good. But doing fast-paced runs (standing while pedaling as fast as you can), which was de rigueur at first, is not. Today, conventional wisdom is to stay seated while doing fast runs. To add intensity, lift your butt a tiny bit off the saddle for a few seconds. For hill climbs and slow jogs, use heavy resistance, stand up, and hold the front of the handlebars, keeping your hips back over the saddle to work your core (abdominals), legs, and butt.

Follow the beat. A good music mix can be the difference between a fun ride and one in which you're simply going through the motions. When a song comes on that I love, my motivation increases along with my stride and heart rate. I prefer songs with lyrics, and if you sing along with the music, you know that you are breathing regularly. If you prefer riding solo, plug in your ear buds, and take your own ride.

Lift Weights—Lift Your Mood

Whether you're buff or the physical equivalent of tone deaf, weight-bearing exercise can help you get or stay fit and sculpted while helping to boost your mood. One way that strength training gives us a mental lift is by restoring some of the dexterity we lose as we get older (such as being able to open a jar or pick up our grandchildren), which can boost our confidence and open up a world of new options for pleasurable activities. It can also alleviate dependence on others and a fear of falling (some might recall being both amused and terrified by the original "I've fallen and I can't get up" TV commercial).

Strength training, especially when mixed with cardio workouts, is also helpful if you are battling mild to moderate depression. One study of sixty older adults with depression found that high-intensity strength training was more effective at reducing depressive symptoms than low-intensity strength training, so work your way up to challenging weights, and keep working out regularly. Combining exer-

cise with therapy can be even more helpful if you are dealing with serious depression.

A Weight Off Your Shoulders

Shrinking muscles can also be reversed through strength
training, which is especially important for women, who are
vulnerable to osteoporosis and need to maintain bone density. Weight lifting might not give you the same cardio boost
of a run or spin, but doing repetitions with free weights or
barbells, which can be done at home or at a gym (ask one of
those bored-looking trainers to spot you), will increase your
heart rate and metabolism.

Do intervals of twelve repetitions for twenty minutes,
stopping in between to rest, every other day. Beginners
should start with light weights and work their way up as
they get stronger. It's important to leave forty-eight hours
between strength training sessions because your muscles
need time to rest so you avoid injuries. You can also spread
out your twenty-minute lifts throughout the day if time is
an issue—it's just as effective as doing it all at once. Here are
some other ideas to pump you up.

Newbies can start by doing push-ups against a wall.
Move to a mat, and get on your knees, keeping your butt
level. As you get stronger, try holding a plank, which is staying in a push-up position with your back flat and butt level
for thirty seconds (on your hands or forearms), increasing
your time gradually. Holding a plank position for five minutes is intense core and strength conditioning even though
you're not moving.

Use free weights (start as light as two pounds, and work
your way up to heavier weights) for bicep curls (forward arm
bends, elbows next to but not touching your sides) and tricep extensions (hold weights in both hands over your head
and lowering them toward the middle of your back, elbows

next to your ears but not touching). Tricep lifts help prevent that unsightly flag waving sometimes known as "lunch lady arms" (apologies to those hard-working women in the cafeteria). You can also use resistance bands, which are light and inexpensive. Get a DVD if you do not have a trainer to show you the correct form. Work up to doing more repetitions each day, week, or month depending on your health and fitness level. Staying at the same level without adding weight will not make any real change in your body or strength.

What's Rafi's Racket?

It requires a heap of upper body strength to serve a ball at a hundred miles per hour across a tennis net, so twenty-eight-year-old champion Rafael Nadal of Spain works his guns by using resistance bands, pulling with one hand across his body from front to back. These bands are used by many athletes such as baseball and volleyball players because they are more portable than weights and they allow for variable resistance and a better workout if used correctly. The bands also work the shoulder and rotator cuff more effectively than free weights.

The bottom line about moving your bottom is this: You can get high on some of your brain's natural chemicals while lowering your risk of developing illnesses such as diabetes and heart disease, so why not put that advice in your pipe and smoke it. Moving the body revitalizes us emotionally and spiritually as well as physically. In the next chapter we'll take revitalization to the next level and explore additional proven practices that also reduce stress and pain and enhance the enjoyment of life with Pleasure Principle #2: Restore.

Pleasure Principle #2

Restore

Revitalizing Mind, Body, and Spirit

Everybody needs beauty as well as bread,
places to play in and pray in, where nature may heal
and give strength to body and soul.

—John Muir, American naturalist

The Bible advises us to restore our souls. Restoring and revitalizing your mind, body, and spirit can involve a variety of activities, including yoga, meditation, prayer, massage, acupuncture (and other complementary practices), eating healthfully, getting enough sleep, taking work breaks, nature walks, and having sex. In this wired age of overstimulation, it also requires making time to unplug. The chatter that continuously pours into our heads makes us *think* that we are connecting to others (it's called social media, after all), but we are actually making virtual connections while we are often bodily and spiritually screened off from the rest of the world.

According to a 2011 University of California study, on any typical day, we take in approximately 174 newspapers' worth of information, five times as much as we did in 1986. There are 21,274 TV stations producing 85,000 hours of original programming each day (as of 2003—undoubtedly more by now), and we watch an average of 5 hours of TV a day. And for every hour of YouTube videos you watch, there are nearly 6,000 hours of new videos being posted.

So how do we transform this overstimulation into rejuvenation? The following activities have been scientifically proven to help us slow down, elevate our mood, reduce our anxiety, and chill without taking a pill.

Meditate—Don't Medicate

In a world rife with quick fixes, magic pills, crash diets, and get-rich-quick schemes, it's nice to know there is a scientifically proven practice that *can* truly change your life (or at least produce dramatic effects) in as little as twenty minutes a day. Yogis and researchers agree: meditating—even for just a few minutes of deep breathing—relaxes the brain, reduces anxiety, and decreases depression. Scores of studies continue to show that the ancient practice of meditation can also help with pain and insomnia, and there's increasing evidence that it can even prevent some diseases by boosting the immune system. That's a whole lot of benefits in exchange for just sitting still and breathing. Long-time meditators have also shown improved brain function resulting from a firing up of neurons, and this increased activity in the prefrontal cortex is associated with positive emotions such as happiness.

Scientists found that after an eight-week course of meditation parts of a participant's brain associated with compassion and self-awareness grew, while parts associated with stress shrank. Stress, which is one of the common reasons people turn to alcohol and other drugs for relief, not only takes a toll on our emotional and mental well-being but also affects our physical health in a variety of ways.

Meditation reduces stress by quieting the constant internal and external prattling in our heads. It can be as simple as sitting quietly and focusing on your breath or a mantra (a meaningful word or phrase). There are numerous traditions and no right way to meditate, so you should find a practice that works for you and stick with it. One of the hardest things about meditation, at least for me, is developing the discipline to do it on a regular basis. But, like exercise, the more you do it the better you will feel. When you first start, pay attention to the changes in your mood or attitude during the day. Do you have more patience? Do you feel more grounded and better able to respond to stressful situations? Are you more in touch with your gut feelings? If so, then you are enjoying some of the many benefits of meditation.

"Yogis and scientists like me have discovered that, in addition to being a great physical exercise, yoga and meditation are antidotes to the stress of modern living," says Sat Bir Singh Khalsa, a Harvard neuroscientist who specializes in yoga research. "By combining physical postures and exercises, breath regulation, deep relaxation and meditation, we literally shift the balance of our stress regulation systems in our brain and our body. Practicing yoga affects the activity of our genes, lowers our heart rate and blood pressure, and decreases the production of 'stress' hormones, which results in lower symptoms of mental and physical distress." The science behind the magic of meditation is that it lowers production of the stress hormone cortisol, which is why meditators are better able to adapt to stress in their lives.

Leah, Age Fifty-Five,
Yoga Teacher from New Jersey
Yoga not only helps with my depression and anxiety, it helps with my physical pain. As soon as I walk into

the yoga studio, whether I'm teaching or practicing, my pain is gone. I don't know why it works, but it does. When I started doing yoga, I was heavily on pain medication. I was always asking my doctor for prescriptions. I'd put my arm in a sling and go to the doctor asking for the Percocet. The yoga got me off the pills. Emotionally yoga clears my blockages, including my anxiety that clutters my mind. When you're doing yoga you are clearing and cleansing your body and your mind. There's also a spiritual element to it. My husband even hears me saying, "God help me," during the day. I realize that what I'm asking for is divine intervention.

Relaxing Forges Stronger Relationships

Ironically, while meditation requires us to look inward, it also helps us to connect with others in more meaningful ways. When couples counselors ask clients to meditate as part of their treatment, for example, they find that their patients become less angry, more self-reflective, and more loving. By becoming more aware of—and honoring—our connection with other people, we are better able to change our preconceptions and see ourselves and our worries in a completely different light. Meditation allows us to embrace and honor our relationships with other people and feel grateful for what is good and loving in our lives.

Yoga and meditation are now being used to treat addictive behaviors, like drug misuse, overeating, and gambling, that cut us off from other people and our sense of a higher power. When Yogi Bhajan started teaching kundalini yoga in the United States during the seventies, he discovered that people were feeling high naturally without the use of mood-altering substances. Bhajan realized that substance abuse is a manifestation of a larger issue. Alcohol, drugs, and even food addiction are just symptoms of a larger emptiness inside. He believes that people with addictions have a spiritual disconnection—they feel lost and empty.

Humans are social creatures with a longing to be part of something and to fit in. If people feel alienated and disassociated, which drugs and alcohol can fuel, that's painful. It's about how you see yourself and your environment. Here's how Yogi Bhajan describes his meditation philosophy:

> Yoga and meditation infuses us with the breath of life. It sustains and maintains us on a daily, moment-to-moment basis. When a rich man is on his death bed with all his money and power, what is he gasping for? Breath—the most important thing in the beginning and the most important thing in the end. In between we forget how important that breath of life is. When that goes, we're done. We are humbled by this. So when you remember your breath you will feel that connection from within. When you forget that, you feel alone.
>
> We don't believe in dwelling on the past. We bless our past, whatever it is, the good and the bad, and then let it go. At best it brought you to a place where you can heal. Blame and shame are heavy loads to carry around. What's important is learning how to let your pain go and replace it with good positive tools and techniques for everyday living. Every day we have to put ourselves back together again and replenish our spiritual vitality and remember who we belong to and who we are connected to.
>
> Yoga is not just about postures. I can stand on my head for two hours or fast for days and still be a jerk. It's about working with the energy within our

bodies, which affects our decisions. Thanks to yoga and meditation, I strive to live each day with grace, integrity and strength.

Randy, Age Fifty-Four, Nursing Student from New Mexico

I used drugs like cocaine, pills, and pot in my early twenties, but started using heroin after marrying a user. I had a good childhood, and my family wasn't alcoholics or drug addicts—I simply used to have fun. I was having seizures since I was a teenager, and the heroin helped calm me down. I wasn't a typical heroin user because I didn't hang around with a drug crowd. I bought, took it home, and used it. I needed to hide it from my straight friends. I spent $100 a day on heroin at one point.

I was high functioning, and I was able to use it and keep my jobs—not that I was a great worker, but I never got fired for using drugs. My family knew I was using, so I finally got to the point where I knew I needed to stop—for them and for health reasons. I tried all kinds of rehabs and counselors, none of which worked. I went to free clinics, expensive ones, therapists, psychiatrists, and even a hospital detox, but nothing stuck.

My turnaround happened when one of my psychologists sent me to a yoga center in 1991. I was ready to be locked up and treated like I had been at other rehabs, and I was planning my escape, but this was different. I was tired of rehashing the same old stuff. I had done some yoga, but I had never done meditation before. Meditation helped me find my higher self. I recognized emotions and feelings for what they were, and I learned how to deal with them and let them go. I understood that my negative reactions were fleeting, that I didn't have to be guided by them. I was careful not to get overstimulated or get overly sad. I recognized my strength, beauty, and potential.

I meditate regularly and try to keep my focus and balance by doing yoga, which helps my body stay healthy. Whenever I'm feeling stress, I go to my office and meditate. I learned to have better control and to feel good without drugs.

Meditation can be done anywhere. You do not need to be in a yoga studio, a dark room, or even a quiet space in order to meditate, although these things do help. You can also try guided meditation (search online to find a place near you) or find a teacher who can instruct you in a class setting or one-on-one.

Just Breathe: A Basic Breathing Meditation
Because breathing is an integral part of yoga and meditation, learning how to control your breath will help you focus and calm your mind. Try this exercise.

Sit with a straight spine, head erect, and chin slightly tucked in. Begin long, slow, deep breathing through your nose. As you inhale, your abdomen (belly) should extend as though it is being filled up with air like a balloon. As you continue to inhale, your chest might also expand and your shoulders rise. As you start to exhale, the chest contracts first. As the exhale continues, your abdomen will pull in as though it is being squeezed like an accordion. Your breath should be steady and smooth at four breaths per minute or slower (fifteen seconds or longer for each breath), if possible.

Remember, it is important to breathe through your nose and not the mouth. Your eyes should be closed during this exercise, and your attention focused only on the flow of your breath. Your focus can be on the sound of your breath, the temperature of the air as it enters your nostrils, or the movement of your chest and abdomen. The more you keep your attention on your breath, the more you will feel yourself becoming relaxed. If your attention wanders, which happens frequently, especially to beginners, patiently bring your attention back to your breath. Let your thoughts pass through your mind without comment. Continue for three minutes or longer.

The Relaxation Response

While meditation is an ancient practice, the Relaxation Response (RR), which also produces feelings of calm and well-being, was discovered by Harvard researcher Dr. Herbert Benson in the seventies. It is a simple technique that can be done while meditating, doing yoga or tai chi, or praying, but it can also be done while running or even when standing in line at the supermarket. You don't have to go to a quiet room, lie still, or even close your eyes, but the fewer distractions the better, especially for beginners. With practice you will be able to calm your mind regardless of where you are or what is going on around you. Here's how to do the RR, according to Benson:

1. Select a word, sound, mantra, prayer, or thought that you find soothing and peaceful. Repeat the word or phrase, and focus your mind in the moment.

2. When other thoughts, sounds, or distractions intrude, let them go, and concentrate once again on step 1. Don't worry if you have random thoughts at first. Just acknowledge them, and let them pass through your mind. Some people like to imagine butterflies flying out of the top of their head or bubbles floating away. Whatever works for you is fine.

Mindfulness meditation, which has been shown to help people with everything from addiction to post-traumatic stress disorder (PTSD), is similar to RR except for the mantra, which is replaced by attention to the intake and outflow of breath.

Because our minds are so active, one of the hardest parts of mastering the RR is learning how to control your thoughts and focus on your word, thought, or phrase. Clearing your mind is like rebooting your computer: it allows you to recharge and makes you feel better in the long run. Doing the Relaxation Response will help you to relieve your anxiety and can even prevent stress.

Benson's research in mind-body medicine found that doing twenty minutes of RR for eight weeks altered the white blood cells (the ones that help our body fight off infections and some cancers) in participants. While scientists are still not exactly sure why RR works, reducing the stress in our lives can help us fend off disease and addictions.

Spirituality

Incorporating spirituality into your life does not necessarily require going to a house of worship, although organized religion does give many people great comfort. Spirituality isn't just about sermons and services; it's about having a connection with something bigger than ourselves. It's about understanding the true meaning and purpose in our lives. It's about finding inner peace.

"Our emotions and our moods are the cornerstones of our well-being in terms of how we perceive and interact with the world," says Elaine Ferguson, a Chicago-based holistic doctor and author of *SuperHealing: Engaging Your Mind, Body, and Spirit to Create Optimal Health and Well-Being.* "My experience with patients is that they are not connected with their spirituality and emotions. They don't incorporate it into their daily lives. Something is missing. When people love themselves they don't need all these chemical mood elevators to make them feel good. Love is what I call one of the 'emotional supernutrients' along with joy, peace, creativity, enthusiasm. All these things are the essence of our spirit and they are what most of us are searching for."

As Ferguson points out, and as nearly all religions tell us, people need to nourish their souls. This is why we must set aside some time, at least one day a week, but ideally more, for spiritual reflection. Because so many of us carry our smartphones with us at all times, work follows us everywhere. Rabbi Steven Leder, author of *More Money Than God: Living a Rich Life without Losing Your Soul,* explains how the ancient rabbis thought of the Sabbath as living a seventh of your life in heaven. By observing the Sabbath, he said, we are calling a truce in the battle for economic existence that most of us wage during the week. Giving ourselves a day of rest is a way of reclaiming our life.

> To me, the Sabbath is about having time alone in my prayers to God, a poem, a song, a walk holding my wife's soft hand, or spending time with my children. "For others it could be about pruning roses, listening to a Brahms concerto, having a sumptuous meal, or taking a long nap. Some people mistakenly believe the Sabbath is about sloth. But it takes a great deal of discipline to observe the Sabbath because it means we must clear a path during the other days of the week for this special day. I guarantee that if we took the Sabbath as seriously as we take our jobs, we would lead far richer lives. I understand that observing the Sabbath is one of the hardest things to do, but once you start reclaiming this day for yourself, you will never go back.

**Parisnicole Payton, Age Forty-Five,
Sports and Entertainment Publicist from Pennsylvania**
My career is extremely stressful. I work long hours
providing public relation services to A-list clients who
are extremely demanding. There are times I go weeks
without sleep. I had to make a commitment not to work
on Sunday. I needed time to recharge. On Sunday, I
attend church and meditate. This helps me to eliminate
stress, recharge, and prepare myself physically and
mentally for the upcoming week. If you want to improve
your mental strength, take two steps back in order to
actively and productively move forward. You must listen
to your inner voice that tells you to slow down, relax,
and rest. By taking care of your mind, body, and spirit,
you will achieve a natural high.

Touch, Sex, and Stress

Studies show that physical contact can help lower our stress,
so reach out and touch someone you love today. When asked
about this in an email interview, Amanda Itzkoff, a New
York–based psychiatrist wrote, "Hugging is said to reduce
blood pressure, while kissing releases chemicals that are
known to eliminate stress hormones." She explained that
having sex produces oxytocin, a "pro-social" hormone that
floods a person's brain immediately after orgasm. "Elevated
levels of oxytocin are linked with a greater sense of trust and
reduced perceptions of threat, in addition to lower levels of
cortisol, the stress hormone," Itzkoff says. "This combination creates feelings of pleasure, contentment and trust."

Still, our desire for sex can wane, depending on our
physical health and life's circumstances. When we have had
a particularly stressful week, are the caretakers of young,
demanding children or ailing partners or older parents, or
are aging ourselves, our sex drive can plummet. Still, while

stress can have a hand in lowering our libido, sex can also be a great stress reliever, which is why we often fall into a peaceful slumber after climaxing (far healthier than the postcoitus cigarette back in the day). The following research supports why we should try to maintain an active sex life and why sex will always rank at the top of the Pleasure Principle list.

Good Sex, Better Mood

In an Arizona State University study of fifty-eight middle-aged women, researchers found that sex and physical intimacy led participants to feel less stressed and be in a better mood the next day. Interestingly, these results were not found when women had orgasms without a partner, which shows that emotional intimacy, particularly for women, might be just as important as physical intimacy. The same study also found that being less stressed often leads to having more sex. (Duh!) It doesn't take a study to understand that when we are feeling less anxious (or at least in a better mood), we are more likely to desire and engage in more sex.

Another study examined subjects' blood pressure while speaking in public or doing challenging math problems—situations that tend to make most of us anxious. Researchers found that those who had recently had sex tended to have either lower baseline blood pressures, less of a blood pressure rise during stressful events, or both. The conclusion: having sex can lead to feeling less stressed during (or perhaps before) engaging in challenging situations.

Paulo Coelho,
in *Manuscript Found in Accra: A Novel*
If two bodies merely join together, that is not sex, it is merely pleasure. Sex goes far beyond pleasure. In sex,

relaxation and tension go hand in hand, as do pain and pleasure, shyness and the courage to go beyond one's limits. How can such opposing states exist in harmony? There is only one way: by surrendering yourself. Because the act of surrender means: "I trust you." It isn't enough to imagine everything that might happen if we allowed ourselves to join not just our bodies, but our souls as well. . . . Allowing someone else to make us happy will make them happy too.

Coming to Our Senses

Sex is not just good for our soul, as Paulo Coelho points out, it is good for our mental and physical health. For one, sex takes our minds off of our troubles (at least in the short term—longer if you are a sexual marathoner.) It also provides some of the following mind and body benefits:

- *Deep breathing.* Like the Relaxation Response and meditation, the heavy breathing we do during sex relaxes the body, oxygenates the blood, and reduces our anxious thoughts and feelings.

- *Endorphins.* Sex is yet another source for those of us who are jonesing for endorphins (i.e., everyone) and other feel-good hormones, which sexual activity releases.

- *Physical workout.* Again, depending on your level of enthusiasm and athleticism, sex can produce the same kind of benefits that you get when exercising.

Sex, like anything that makes us feel good, can be a compulsive activity for some of us. Whether it's with serial partners or Internet porn, compulsive sex has the opposite effect from connecting us with others and creating intimacy. Professional help and Twelve Step support groups are recommended if you think the high of sex is as addictive for you like the high of cocaine is for others.

Get More Sleep

While you might not consider sleep a high, consider how good you feel when you're really rested and how hung over you feel when you're not. Most Americans are not getting enough sleep, studies show, which puts enormous stress on our bodies and minds. Insomnia disorder is defined as at least three months of poor sleep, causing problems at work, at home, and in relationships. Getting enough restorative sleep is vital for reducing depression, which affects some eighteen million Americans in any given year. And most of these people suffer from insomnia.

There has been some recent debate about the "right" amount of zzzs necessary for people to function properly during the day. Eight hours for adults used to be the magic number, but the National Sleep Foundation now says that not only do different age groups need different amounts of sleep, but just like other characteristics we are born with, the amount of sleep we need to function well may differ from person to person. While you may be at your absolute best sleeping seven hours a night, others might clearly need nine hours to live a happy, productive life. Sleeping long enough to go through four or five REM (rapid eye movement) cycles is probably the best measure for how long you should sleep. This is when you're dreaming the dreams you're most likely to remember, which can sometimes rival LSD for a trippy experience. (But at least if it's a bad trip, all you have to do to come down is wake up.)

Another reason there is no one-size-fits-all for snoozing is our sleep debt, the accumulated sleep that is lost as a result of poor habits, sickness, inability to shut off and wind down, environmental factors, or other causes. For instance, you might meet your personal requirement for sleep on any given night or a few nights in a row, but still have accumulated sleep debt. We might feel more tired and less alert at certain times, particularly in conjunction with our natural sleep cycles—those times in the twenty-four-hour period when we are biologically programmed to be more sleepy and less alert, such as mid-afternoon.

Taking breaks is biologically restorative, but naps are even better (and are not just for babies and elders). In several studies, a nap of even ten minutes helped improve brain function and decreased fatigue while reducing stressful cortisol levels. Parents know the importance of creating a sleep routine for getting kids to bed on time—the same goes for grown-ups. Going to bed and waking up at the same time is one way to create a sleep ritual.

To help you sleep, drink a hot cup of decaffeinated tea, listen to soothing music, burn some incense (lavender is said to have a calming effect), or do a little light reading before bedtime. Make sure your bedroom is as dark as possible, with no ambient light from phones, computers, or TVs.

You Knead It

Massages do more than soothe sore muscles. A growing body of research suggests that a rubdown reduces cortisol and lowers our blood pressure—yet another natural way to help lift our spirits and stave off depression. Massage has also been shown to boost those anxiety-busting neurotransmitters serotonin and dopamine.

If you've ever dozed off on a massage table, you know firsthand(s) that a massage can promote restorative sleep. A number of studies chalk this up to massage's affect on delta waves, those brain waves connected to deep sleep, according to *Health* magazine. And, like muscle and back pain, tension headaches can also be alleviated after a massage. A 2009 study found that a thirty-minute massage decreased pain for people with tension headaches and even curbed some of the stress and anger associated with that pounding head. Because of all these benefits, massage can also be helpful for people living with or undergoing treatment for serious illnesses, including cancer, by relieving fatigue, pain, and nausea.

DIY Massage

Professional massages can be costly, especially if you live in a big city, so if you can't afford the full wrapped-in-a-towel monty, I recommend a ten-minute chair massage (done fully clothed and available at many nail salons for around $10 plus tip) and a pedicure, which includes a five-minute foot massage for between $20 and $30, or giving yourself a rubdown (free). I'm not talking about masturbation, here—which belongs in a previous section and is also a good stress reliever—but rather a relaxing, tension-melting muscle massage that can be done anywhere—even in your office during your lunch hour (close the door, and try not to moan too loudly).

According to Sandhiya Ramaswamy, there is no greater expression of self-love than anointing oneself from head to toe with warm oil. You can buy aromatic massage oils online (try mountainroseherbs.com) or at your local health food store. These special oils are used to enrich the massage experience with therapeutic botanical properties. It is believed that those who are massaged with oil become saturated with love. The following are Ramaswamy's exact instructions for a DIY massage.

Steps for Self-Massage

- Warm the oil (pour approximately ¼ cup into a mug and warm using a coffee-cup warmer). Test the temperature by putting a drop on your inner wrist, oil should be comfortably warm and not hot.

- Sit or stand comfortably in a warm room.

- Apply oil first to the crown of your head and work slowly out from there in circular strokes—spend a couple of minutes massaging your entire scalp (home to many other vital energy points).

- Massage your face in circular motion, including your forehead, temples, cheeks, and jaws (always moving in a upward movement). Be sure to massage your ears, especially your ear-lobes, which has essential nerve endings.

- Use long strokes on the limbs (arms and legs) and circular strokes on the joints (elbows and knees). Always massage toward the direction of your heart.

- Massage the abdomen and chest in broad, clockwise, circular motions. On the abdomen, follow the path of the large intestine; moving up on the right side of the abdomen, then across, then down on the left side.

- Finish the massage by spending at least a couple of minutes massaging your feet. Feet are a very important part of the body with the nerve endings of essential organs and vital marma points.

- Sit with the oil for 5–15 minutes if possible so that the oil can absorb and penetrate into the deeper layers of the body.

- Enjoy a warm bath or shower. You can use a mild soap on the "strategic" areas, avoid vigorously soaping and rubbing the body.

- When you get out of the bath, towel dry gently. Blot the towel on your body instead of rubbing vigorously.

- After your self-massage, enjoy the feeling of having nourished your mind, body, and spirit, and try to keep that high with you throughout your day.

ACUPUNCTURE GETS TO THE POINT

Acupuncture is the stimulation of specific points along the body using thin needles or the application of heat, pressure, or laser light. An ancient Chinese practice, it is used to treat a range of conditions, including back pain, headaches, and digestive problems. It is also being used successfully for depression and addiction to drugs, alcohol, and nicotine.

Acupuncture works by correcting imbalances in the body's natural flow of energy through channels known as meridians; it does not always involve being stuck like a porcupine with numerous needles. Eastern practitioners believe the body is made up of different channels, so stimulating points along these channels (there are over four hundred acupuncture points all over the body) helps balance or correct any deficiencies or blockages. Research using MRIs has shown that when you place a needle at certain acupuncture points, areas of the brain light up. The stimulated areas that are associated with our emotions release a flood of endorphins and dopamine that act as painkillers and mood enhancers. Acupuncture has been used to treat the cravings associated with addiction to nicotine, opiates, and other drugs.

Jadran from California says, "I started acupuncture for my anxiety/stress issues, which stemmed from having a strict upbringing and a number of disturbing issues such as going to war, losing a loved one, and moving from place to place, which left me feeling emotionally drained. Even though I did tai chi and yoga, my problem turned out to be an inability to release tightness of certain deeper muscles in my lower back caused by stress. It can take some time for it to start working, as we can accumulate tightness in our bodies for a lifetime. I always make sure that I'm good to myself and that if any emotions surface after an acupuncture session, I try to accept them and fully let them go."

Rocky Mountain High

In every walk with nature one receives more than he seeks.

—John Muir, American naturalist

Reconnecting with nature is encouraged by just about every religious and philosophical belief system, and science has also proven that we are happiest when we're outdoors. Several studies have shown that a walk in nature can trigger the mind-wandering mode that acts as a reset button in our brains.

In 2005, Richard Louv, cofounder and chairman emeritus of the Children & Nature Network and author of *The Nature Principle: Reconnecting with Life in a Virtual Age*, coined the term "nature-deficit disorder" to describe the growing gap between people and the environment. According to Louv, a nature deficit, like malnutrition, has its consequences. In his book he asks: "What would our everyday lives be like if we were as immersed in nature as we are in technology?"

Research confirms a link between the amount of time we spend in nature, or in homes and workplaces with nature-based designs, and a reduction of stress and depression, a faster healing process, and less need for pain medication if injured. Health care professionals are starting to take notice. In 2010, a pilot program in Portland, Oregon, began pairing physicians with park professionals, who helped children and families get their quotient of nature or, as Louv calls it, their "vitamin N."

Other benefits of vitamin N include enhanced use of our senses and higher work productivity. In 2008, University of Michigan researchers demonstrated that, after just an hour interacting with nature, memory performance and attention spans improved by 20 percent. In April 2014, researchers at the University of Kansas reported a 50 percent boost in creativity for people who spent a few days in nature.

If you would like to enjoy these green benefits (and help keep our environment from disappearing), I suggest trying the any of the following.

Plant a garden. Create a backyard wildlife habitat or plant a vegetable garden from which you can reap what you sow. Grow flowers that will encourage butterflies and birds to flutter by. Bring the great outdoors inside by decorating your home with freshly cut flowers and plants.

Be a nature mentor. Encourage the next generation (your children or grandchildren or other children in your life) to put down the devices and go outside to build forts and other shelters, collect leaves or sea shells (if you live near a beach), observe insects in the backyard, or identify local birds. A small pile of dirt or leaves is all they need for hours of creative playtime.

Start a nature club. Get to know nature where you live by taking regular nature walks with your neighbors, friends, or family. If you are in a city, go to the park, or take a field trip out of town to escape the concrete jungle. As the aptly named motivational speaker Earl Nightingale put it, "Our environment, the world in which we live and work, is a mirror of our attitudes and expectations."

Participate in a local cleanup. Being part of a green team not only is personally rewarding but helps improve our ecologically challenged earth. If you see trash on the ground or sidewalk, don't walk on by; pick it up, and throw it out.

Reduce, reuse, and recycle. The cartoon construction worker Bob the Builder is right (parents know the guy I'm talking about), when he encourages kids (and us) to recycle as much as possible. We all know about separating our plastics, tins, and papers. (Many grocery stores offer plastic-bag recycling bins, so drop them off the next time you go shopping.) For electronic waste, which is presenting another serious environmental hazard, find out where your local recycling center is, and bring your old computers, monitors, cell phones, and batteries to be properly disposed of or refurbished.

For some, connecting with nature is a grander version of connecting with the people and animals in your life—you get outside of your small ego and all its problems and feel a part of something bigger than yourself. That's the message of Pleasure Principle #3: Connect.

Pleasure Principle #3

Connect

Bonding with Family, Friends, and Community

Having an active social life in which you surround yourself with friends and family is one of the most important Pleasure Principles. Studies have shown that feeling a part of a family, circle of friends, and community (e.g., workplace, religious, social, or political group) throughout our lifetime helps stave off depression and, of course, loneliness, while keeping our minds vibrant. There is some evidence that spending time with others can even increase our longevity.

Our closest bonds are usually with our immediate family and friends. If we were raised in a stable home environment with at least one caretaker who showed us love and nurtured our sense of self-worth, we had a better chance of forming healthy relationships during childhood, adolescence, and adulthood.

With that foundation, we're more likely as adults to find compatible partners and create an atmosphere of trust that carries over into building our own family. It also helps us bond with coworkers, should we have them, and grow our circle of social relationships. This network of connections with a variety of people helps us move beyond focusing on only our own needs and wants to identifying with a larger community that strengthens our sense of self.

When this extends into our religious or spiritual life, it also helps define our moral center and gives our lives purpose. This has been universally true across history and cultures, with family and tribal identity providing a healthy sense of self and purpose to not only humans but also other social animals like wolves, dogs, elephants, and our closer genetic relatives, the great apes. The need to connect is literally in our chromosomes.

If we don't receive the nurture we need in childhood, and especially if we were abused or have a predisposition to develop a mental health disorder (including addiction), we often develop a lack of trust in ourselves and others as adults, and find it difficult to build that network of family, friends, and community that provides the support and sense of well-being necessary for a fulfilling life. We're more likely to turn to mood-altering drugs, compulsive sex, gambling, and other addictive behaviors to create a false sense of contentment that is missing in our everyday lives. One reason that Twelve Step peer recovery programs have been successful is that addicts learn to mend their broken connections to the people in their lives, which produces a healing of their spirit and provides them with the pleasures and highs that come with giving and receiving care and help from others.

SOCIALIZING CAN BE CHALLENGING
IF YOU CAN'T DRINK

Of course, socializing can be difficult for many people who have depended on "social lubricants" in the past to help ease the anxiety of meeting new people. If these kinds of get-togethers present too much temptation to get tipsy, work on making your social circle consist of only those people you feel comfortable with, or decline invitations to cocktail parties and other events where there is the possibility that many of the guests might be getting looped. Or, if you attend, have a plan for dealing with your triggers for drinking or using; for example, connect with other people who aren't drinking, have your sponsor's number handy, and have an escape plan if things get too difficult. You might have to change your social circle to include more people who indulge in healthful activities if you are used to hanging with a crowd that parties hard. There are plenty of ways to socialize without drugs and alcohol, and this chapter will provide a host of ideas to choose from.

The Roseto Study

In his best seller *Outliers*, Malcolm Gladwell writes about the groundbreaking study of a group of Italian immigrants who lived in Roseto, Pennsylvania, named for the small village south of Rome from which they came. As Gladwell and the author Elaine Ferguson both point out, in the fifties, when the study was done, steak and potatoes were the staple of most American diets, and scotch, martinis, and cigarettes were as ubiquitous as billboards on the highway. Cholesterol-lowering drugs such as Lipitor and heart disease awareness campaigns had not yet emerged. It was a time when heart attacks were the leading cause of death in men under the age of sixty-five.

Elaine R. Ferguson, Chicago-based
holistic medical practitioner and author
of *SuperHealing: Engaging Your Mind, Body,*
and *Spirit to Create Optimal Health and Well-Being*

When I was in college I learned that monkey and human babies can be given all the physical ingredients that they need to survive, but if they don't receive love they become severely depressed and withdrawn. This is not just true for babies, but for adults as well. We need to be in relationships and to be a part of a community so we can share with others. We are tribal people, so this is critical to our survival. Having a social circle is also good for our physical health. One of the most fascinating studies I came across was conducted in the fifties and called the Roseto Study, which found that participants who were doing all the wrong things in terms of preventing heart disease (smoking, eating fatty foods, not exercising) didn't get heart disease because they had such a strong sense of community. Human beings need to be in relationships with others because it's what makes our lives rich.

Stewart Wolf, a physician who taught at the University of Oklahoma and spent his summers in Roseto, discovered a medical mystery. He enlisted some of his students and colleagues on a quest to find out why there were so few heart attacks among the dozen or so Rosetans. The researchers pored over the death certificates going back as far as they could, analyzed physicians' records, took medical histories, and constructed family genealogies. The results were astonishing.

"In Roseto, virtually no one under fifty-five died of a heart attack, or showed any signs of heart disease. For men over sixty-five, the death rate from heart disease in Roseto was roughly half that of the United States as a whole," Gladwell writes. Wolf brought in sociologists to help with his investigation. "There was no suicide, no alcoholism, no drug addiction, and very little crime. There was no one on welfare. No peptic ulcers. These people were dying of old age. That's it."

It was, as Gladwell's book title suggests, an "outlier" town.

Perhaps you are wondering if the much-lauded Mediterranean diet accounted for these overwhelmingly healthy citizens. Nope. The Rosetans, it turns out, were cooking with lard, instead of the much healthier Italian staple, olive oil. The typical Rosetan's eating habits consisted of a whopping 41 percent of calories from fat. Nor was this a town where people took brisk hikes like their goat-herding ancestors, or got up at dawn to run ten miles on a tree-lined trail. On the contrary, the Pennsylvanian Rosetans smoked heavily, and many were overweight.

If it wasn't the diet and exercise that kept these people healthy, then, Wolf wondered, might it be genetics? The Rosetans were a close-knit group from the same region of Italy, so maybe they were products of a particularly hardy stock whose genes protected them from disease. Wolf proceeded to track down relatives of the Rosetans who were living in other parts of the United States to see if they had the same remarkable good health as their cousins in Pennsylvania. Again, the answer was no.

He then examined the Eastern Pennsylvanian region where the Rosetans lived. Was it possible that there was something in water or soil that contained healthful properties? The nearby towns, Bangor and Nazareth, just a few miles away, were populated with the same number of hardworking European immigrants. Wolf combed through both towns' medical records. For men over sixty-five, the death rates from heart disease in Nazareth and Bangor were something like three times that of Roseto. Another brick wall.

What Wolf eventually concluded was that the secret of Roseto's vigor wasn't diet or exercise or genes or even the region itself. The answer lay in the way these Rosetans lived. Families visited each other; men and women stopped to chat on the street; they cooked for one another in their backyards. Many homes had three generations living under one roof, and grandparents were treated with respect rather than derision for their advanced age or frailties. They went to church regularly, which had a calming, unifying effect. There were no less than twenty-two civic organizations in a town of just under two thousand people. The townspeople also discouraged the wealthier residents (not that there were many) from flaunting their success and helped the less fortunate improve their circumstances.

The Rosetans were healthy because they were a close-knit, social people. The transplanted *paesani* culture of southern Italy created a nurturing, protective social cocoon of sorts, where caring for one's neighbor inoculated people from the debilitating stress and pressures of the modern world. When John G. Bruhn, a fellow researcher who was brought in by Wolf to work on the study, visited Roseto for the first time, he saw large, home-cooked family meals and bakeries; people walking up and down the street, sitting on their porches chatting; the blouse mills where the women worked during the day, while the men worked in the slate quarries. "It was magical," Bruhn said.

When Bruhn and Wolf first presented their findings to the medical community, they were greeted with skepticism. At the convention, their peers presented data, complex charts, and gene analysis, while the Rosetan researchers spoke about the mysterious and miraculous benefits of socializing with friends and living with multigenerational relations. Health is not, as conventional wisdom has it, only about what we eat and how much we exercise, but about how we live. The Roseto study taught us to look at the community we live in, who our friends and families are, and the values that guide our everyday lives. This begs the question, decades after this study was conducted: Why have so many of us forgotten this vital Pleasure Principle?

Learning from Girl Power

Nearly every modern era has its powerful women's groups, which come in all stripes—from the genteel sewing circles and politically charged suffragettes, to the tool-toting World War II riveters, League of Women Voters, and National Organization for Women. Today we can add soccer moms, Mocha Moms, feminist bloggers, and women who are "leaning in" and having more influence in Congress and the corporate suite.

We can often take the pulse of a generational zeitgeist by looking at the iconic fictional characters in the media, including HBO's well-heeled, zinger-slinging *Sex and the City* ladies who brunch and, most recently, the hip and whip-smart, post–Great Recession characters in Lena Dunham's *Girls*. And while many women of all ages still hang with their childhood and college friends or meet at fundraisers, mommy-and-me classes, children's parties, and PTA meetings, their social circles have now expanded into cyberspace. Skout, an online global social network for meeting new people, recently conducted a survey among more than 3,800 women to uncover the latest trends and habits around women's friendships in today's digital world. Its key findings include:

- *BFs before FWBs.* Fifty-five percent of women say their relationship with a best friend is more important than one with a romantic partner.

- *Friends from childhood will always be special.* Sixty-two percent of women surveyed say one of their closest friends is someone they met as a child.

- *Mobile devices and the Internet are used to stay in touch with close friends.* Eighty-eight percent of women say they communicate with their close friends several times per week using mobile phones or the Internet. (In fact, 53 percent do so every day.)

- *The majority of women have a long lost friend.* Nearly 70 percent of women say they have a good friend they've lost touch with and would like to reconnect with. (Isn't that what Facebook's for?)

- *Stuck on a deserted island, women would prefer to be there with a friend.* More women would choose to be stuck on a deserted island with a friend instead of a significant other, a family member, a beloved pet, or a celebrity. (In the movie *Cast Away*, I believe Tom Hanks made the best of it with a volleyball. Come to think of it, I wouldn't mind being stuck on an island with Tom Hanks.)

- *BFFs can be "Boyfriends Forever."* Thirty-five percent of women say their closest friend is a male.

The moral of this survey: Whatever your gender, if you are so inclined to reach out while reclined with your smartphone or laptop, you can use Facebook, Instagram, Pinterest, Snapchat, Vine, Skout, and other social media to weave a wider web, but don't forget to meet up sometime F2F (face to face).

Enlarge Your Circles

Unlike the sites mentioned above, there is another Internet-based girl group that focuses on moving from screen to being seen, which is optimal when making real relationships. It's called Girlfriend Circles (girlfriendcircles.com), and it's perfect for women who have just moved to a new town, new moms who are feeling isolated and disconnected from their former child-free lifestyle, or those simply seeking to branch out. Here's some information on Girlfriend Circles that includes good advice to everyone regardless of gender for making meaningful connections with friends using social media to create groups around common needs and interests.

Build friendships in small groups. Small talk, handshaking, and networking are not the goals of forming a friendship. The same goes for typing or texting back and forth without actually meeting the person you are writing to. The answer is meeting in small groups, first online and then in person, so you can determine whom you click with the best.

Create Connecting Circles. Connecting Circles is a process by which you build a group of like-minded friends and acquaintances by starting with easy back-and-forth questions so you're not at risk of one person doing all the talking or trying to think up conversation starters. Out of this back-and-forth conversation, compatible groups can naturally form around common interests and personal affinities.

You are in control. Some social clubs are all about one person planning all the events. Girlfriend Circles provides a model for group gatherings that are more like a cooperative in which people can plan and host any event they want, with anyone they want, whenever they want. Group members can attend as many events as they like—or not.

Friendships aren't superficial. The goal is to create friendships that last. This means group members must be consistent with each other so that real friendships can form. (In other words, keep the conversation going.)

Meet up. Group members can meet in Connecting Circles at different cafés around their town or city so they get to try out new places. Events and places listed come from people in the community. (By the way, trying new things is a Pleasure Principle.)

Making Connections:
Let Us Count the Ways

There are as many ways to meet and connect with others as there are people. It depends on your interests and personality; sometimes, you have to find the courage to try new things that can expand your sense of who you are and give you a sense of belonging. This includes developing a scientific spirit: if something doesn't work the first time, learn from that experience and try something else.

Meet-Ups

Meet-ups, which we learned about from Girlfriend Circles, are another increasingly common way for groups of people with shared interests to connect with planned meetings that are posted online. It allows people to form offline clubs in local communities around the world. If you can't find one that interests you, start your own meet-up. Here are just a few of the established interest groups in New York City. Check out the ones in your location:

- Community & Environment
- Fitness
- Singles Volleyball
- Food shows
- Health & Wellbeing
- Yoga
- New Age and Spirituality
- Parents and Families
- Dance

Meetup.com is a site that provides an online resource for staging these gatherings. Just put in your zip code, and get out there!

Book Clubs

As brick-and-mortar bookstores, libraries, and newspapers continue to go the way of the roller rink, people who love to read (and there are millions out there) have taken matters into their own dust- and newsprint-covered hands. They form book clubs, which, like the literary salons of another century, are held in various apartments and houses, usually on weekends or evenings, sometimes accompanied by food and beverages. Books are chosen democratically a month in advance, read, and then discussed. Those of you who have taken English literature classes (also a diminishing number—oh, the humanities!) will be familiar with this deconstructive MO. Discussing your favorite novel or nonfiction book with others is social bonding for the literati.

Keep in mind that a book club doesn't have to be all that literary. You can choose your own genre, including popular novels (romance, science fiction, mystery, fantasy, horror, etc.), various nonfiction categories on topics you're interested in, books that have been made into movies so you can combine watching the film and reading the book, and so on. The important thing is that you read something interesting that sparks discussion, which can lead to other topics—which can eventually lead to connections with like-minded people who can become new friends.

If you don't like to read that much and/or don't know many people who do, you can form a movie group and have a member choose a movie to watch for each meeting, leaving time for discussion and socializing.

Fantasy Sports

Somewhat less heady than a book club, but stimulating another area of the brain that requires math skills by way of statistics, fantasy football (and other sports) is an interactive competition in which users compete against each other as ersatz general managers of fantasy teams built from drafting real players. The teams that you manage are made up of professional players in the National Football League or other sports conference. You are able to draft, trade, add, or drop players, and change rosters every week.

Fantasy football and baseball are nearly as popular as NASCAR, thanks to ESPN Fantasy Sports, CBS, Yahoo! Fantasy Sports, and the NFL itself, which will track statistics online, eliminating the need to check box scores in newspapers regularly. Go online to join or start a league. Leagues are also popular in the workplace these days, and this can be a good way to connect with people you like at work. Compare notes with friends about which players to draft and check out the message boards for fellow faux team managers. Find a big screen (you probably know someone who has a large flat-screen TV on their wall), get out the chips and salsa (or the stale cheese and crackers from your last party), and go to town. You can even make a field trip to an actual stadium. When one season ends, you can start all over with fantasy basketball, hockey, or whatever sport you follow.

The point is to create an environment for sharing your interests with other people and in the course of interacting with them, forge a bond that takes you outside of your own head to experience the pleasure of being part of a group.

Pick-Up Games

If you are more of an active participant than a foam-finger-waving, face-painting, bleacher-sitting fan, suit up and join a pick-up game in your favorite sport. Here's what Brooklyn resident Isaac Eger wrote about his search for a basketball pick-up game in a 2012 essay published in the *New York Times*:

Pickup games generally take place on weekend mornings and weekday evenings after 4 p.m. It is far too hot at midday to run around on the cooked asphalt for a few hours. Finding games at those hours has been incredibly easy. Every day I have set out and I have stumbled upon full-court pickup. In Florida, I would sometimes drive 20 miles to find evidence of a single halfcourt game. In Brooklyn, I check a map, look for green spots, and within half an hour I am sweaty and shooting.

New York ballers do not realize how good they have it. At Red Hook park, as my teammates and I made introductions, they asked me where I was from. I told them I had biked from Bushwick, six miles away.

"You came that far just to play some ball?" They couldn't believe it.

Though everything seems to be less than an hour away, people do not appear too inclined to venture far beyond their neighborhood. Perhaps there is a level of comfort that comes with picking a court and sticking with it—like picking your favorite bar or cigarette. All of the players seem to know one another's nicknames, tricks and extended families. . . .

That is why so many shooters, I suspect, are corn-fed boys from the Midwest and prep schoolers from the suburbs: the country and sprawl quarantine them, and they have nothing to do but practice fundamentals by their lonesome.

There are pick-up games for soccer, baseball, softball, volleyball, and probably lacrosse, especially if you live somewhere more corn dog than hot dog. Go to nextgamenation .com to find a game near you.

This is a great opportunity to practice Pleasure Principles #1 and #3 simultaneously!

Make a BFF
(Best Furry Friend)

Friends come in all shapes, sizes, genders, and breeds. In other words, they don't have to be human. Studies have shown that pets improve our moods and help relieve our stress, which is why pet therapy is widely used in nursing homes and hospitals and with people with special needs to help reduce loneliness, anger, or depression.

Erika Friedmann, an expert in pet therapy research, found that cardiac patients' survival rates are higher for those who owned pets, and that the elderly who have pets made fewer visits to the doctor's office. When research subjects played with their four-legged or feathered friends, they showed a significant decrease in their resting heart rate and blood pressure, as well as positive mood changes.

Researchers have found that interaction with pets—even if they don't belong to you—can reduce anxiety, ease blood pressure and heart rate, and offset feelings of depression for people of all ages. One study showed that exposure to an aviary filled with songbirds lowered depression in elderly men at a veterans' hospital, while another noted the improved moods of depressed college students after they hung out with a therapy dog.

Because a common symptom of depression is feeling isolated, those who love their animal companions know that having a pet can lead to socializing with people. Here's why.

Pets can encourage you to stay active, even if you are feeling depressed. Dogs need to be walked three times a day, so no matter how much you want to crawl into bed with the covers over your head, you must grab that leash and take a canine constitutional. Along the way, you might meet a neighbor who engages you in conversation, or if you go to a dog park, you will see other owners you recognize who might just help lift your flagging spirits. Plus, watching puppies frolicking around is a natural form of entertainment. If you don't believe me, check YouTube for some of the most frequently posted viral videos.

Animals are conversation starters. When people see a cute dog, they are likely to approach you, and might even ask if they can pet it. Make sure your dog is comfortable with being touched by a stranger, and let it smell the person's hand first. If the stranger is offering treats, make sure they are given with an open palm below the chin, especially if you have a rescue dog that is a little skittish. Many a friendship has been formed in a dog park.

Pets provide unconditional love and companionship. One thing you can say for a pet is that they love you no matter what you look like or how much money you make. You are never alone when you have a dog, cat, bird, hamster, or whatever kind of companion you choose. An aquarium can be pleasant to come home to, even if you can't pet your clownfish Nemo.

Therapy Animals

Groups like the American Humane Association and the Delta Society offer animal-assisted therapy programs for people with depression and other mood disorders, including post-traumatic stress disorder. When looking for a pet therapy group in your area, be sure to find out how much training the therapy pets and animal handlers have had. The American Humane Association emphasizes that the good that can come from pet therapy can be undone if the pets are not gentle and well-trained.

For those who are simply looking for the unconditional love we get from our furry friends, I strongly suggest going to your local animal shelters, which are filled to capacity with loving animals in need of a good forever home, and not to pet stores that use inhumane puppy and other mills. If you are looking for a particular breed of dog or cat, first check out the adoption centers to ask if one is available or look online for adoption organizations that specialize in the pedigree you are looking for.

No wild or exotic pets, please! These animals belong in their natural habitat and are probably endangered.

The Six Circles of Hello
(What's Your Friendship Level?)

I have a thirteen-year-old in the throes of puberty who has yet to find a best friend (BF), much to her chagrin, but she does have many acquaintances. I tell her to be patient—it will happen, but friendships often require nurturing, like flowers that need water in order to grow. There are different levels of friendship, of course, depending on your age and stage in life, and they evolve in time from one stage to another—sometimes becoming closer, sometimes moving further apart. Not every friendship will reach BF status, and each relationship is different, which is perfectly normal. Some people might start out as acquaintances and stay that way for a long time before moving to the next stage (or not). Others may develop quickly from online friends to offline friends, and possibly to BFFs (best friends forever). It all depends on how two people click, their expectations, and how much effort they are willing to put into the relationship. Below is one take on the different types of friendship, all of which have their purpose and place in our lives.

Acquaintances

An acquaintance is often called someone you "know in passing," someone you may see and interact with on an occasional or even regular basis, but they are not a real friend. Unless you spend time together outside of whatever circumstance brought you together (work, school, church, political or social club, etc.) you are an acquaintance. The promotion to friendship comes when a relationship develops in which you share personal information and spend more time together. You may be an acquaintance of someone for many years without a true friendship developing. Or it can be the first step to becoming a future friend. It depends on the two people involved and whether or not they click.

Mentor

Mentors are people who share their knowledge and experience with others. It is not unusual for a mentor to be older, and most enjoy helping the mentee by sharing their expertise. Mentors help us navigate our career and personal choices, as well as introduce us to new people. A mentor can become a friend at some point, especially when both people become more like peers on a more or less equal level. It is also possible that a mentor might never be a real friend. They can be, nevertheless, an important part of our lives, and I highly recommend having one.

Casual Friend

A casual friend is someone you have a personal relationship with (you've spent time together and bonded) who can be considered a friend. Your friendships may be slightly different from each other and even include different levels. You may also start out as good friends with someone but then drift back to being occasional friends at some point in your relationship. Friendships are fluid and changing, so it's not unusual to see them go through periods where the people involved feel very close to one another, struggle, drift apart, and then get back together.

Good Friend

A good friend is not necessarily following you on Twitter or on Facebook, or even one of the people on your contact list, but he or she is the go-to person you call when you have a problem or when you want to share a triumph. It's about trust, offering advice, and taking advice. A good friend will listen as much as she or he talks, and ask questions instead of giving monologues (enough about me—what do *you* think about me?). Good friends are people who know the most about your life and have likely been there during the ups and downs. You can have many friends, but as you get older and stop hanging in crews, you are likely to have just a few people you consider good friends, and those are the people you generally see and talk to the most often.

Friends with Benefits (FWBs)

An FWB is usually a casual friend or a good friend (not best friend) you also have sex with when the mood strikes. They are more often than not ex-partners you have stayed close to emotionally as well as sexually.

Best Friends (BFs)

Best friends, also known as BFs, bromances, best buds, or besties, are people you are extremely close to and consider almost as close to as your significant other. They are often people you have known the longest, sometimes since childhood. They are among the *first* people you call when you're excited, hurt, or just want to chat. Best friends can often feel like family because they are there for us during the most important moments in our life. Not everyone has a best friend, and that's okay. Others might have one best friend, which is also fine. Some might have several. It all depends on your personal preference. There is no right way to have relationships—it's about what makes you happy and most comfortable.

Significant Others, Spouses, Family Members

Thousands of books have been written on intimate and family relationships, and it would be hard to do justice to these vital relationships in a paragraph or two. Needless to say, family is where our most important relationships are built, and it is the training ground for learning to reach out to others and give and receive emotional sustenance. A loving relationship with a spouse, child, parent, or grandparent can be the greatest high of all, and if you're going to invest your relationship capital anywhere, this is the place to start. Of course not everyone is married or has a healthy relationship with their family of origin, and perhaps more than anyone, this Pleasure Principle is for them. We need to have the sense of belonging that family gives us, and sometimes that means building our own family of choice from our acquaintances and friends. In addition to the activities we've discussed, this can happen at work, a place of worship, a club (hobby, social, political), a volunteer organization (combining this Pleasure Principle with #6, Give), and so on.

Loneliness

Lonely is the opposite of high. If you're lonely, reach out to someone. If you think you might be depressed, get help. If you know someone who's lonely, be a friend.

Three years ago a woman who lives in my building lost her husband suddenly to a heart attack. Her daughter is in college, so she is living alone in her empty nest. She is a therapist, so she knows a little something about expressing her feelings, but I was taken by surprise one day while riding with her in the elevator making idle chitchat. I made her laugh about something I don't remember, and she turned to me earnestly and said, "Jodie, you are someone I've always liked. It would be great to spend more time with you. I'm really lonely."

I told her that I would love to have her over to my place for coffee or lunch, and we exchanged numbers and emails. Had she not said anything that day, I would not have known the extent of her pain and need for companionship. Sometimes you just have to speak up and tell someone you are lonely. People are generally more than willing to help a friend or neighbor in need.

A great place to meet people is at cultural events, rock concerts, and museums—venues to share our creative spirit. This takes us to Pleasure Principle #4: Create.

Pleasure Principle #4

Create

Expressing and Expanding
the Inner Self

A 2010 university study published in the *American Journal of Public Health* found that music, visual arts therapy, dancing, and creative writing were effective in reducing some physiological and psychological disorders. This Pleasure Principle requires you to stretch your creative muscles by dipping your toes or paintbrush in some of the activities below. Caveat: this means you must stop multitasking and immerse yourself in a single task for between thirty to fifty minutes.

The Healing Power of Music

According to a 2014 Wakefield Research survey of one thousand American adults age eighteen and older, 86 percent prefer aural (listening) pleasures to visual ones in order to relax, and more than one-third of the respondents chose music as a way to help them decompress. Other studies show that listening to music is a great way to improve your attention, build up self-confidence, and develop social skills and a sense of belonging.

The so-called Mozart effect study, which suggested that listening to classical music can boost cognitive performance, has been pretty much debunked (disappointing many an expectant parent who held a radio, Walkman, or iPod to the belly of a pregnant woman hoping that the growing fetus would somehow become smarter in utero). While fetal music might not produce baby Einsteins, playing or listening to music once born does create a good vibe by lowering our blood pressure, activating our brain's reward centers, and depressing the activity in the part of the brain associated with fear and negative emotions. In other words, it reduces stress.

In his book *Musicophilia*, Oliver Sacks writes eloquently about the power of music, which, he says, can "move us to the heights or depths of emotion." Music therapy is increasingly being used in medical settings to soothe premature infants in neonatal units as well as treat depression. There are so many ways to listen to music these days: streaming on your computer, using an MP3 player, or turning on the radio (it helps control road rage—unless you're listening to some of the more incendiary heavy metal or rap). There is no shortage of mobile audio apps that give you unlimited access to millions of songs and turn your smartphone into an ear-bud radio. From Spotify, Pandora, and iTunes to Shazam, there are a lot of options, with new ones coming online every day, for tailoring your music offerings on your laptop, phone, or tablet.

Make Your Own Music

Even more rewarding than passive listening, learning how to play an instrument and maybe even joining a band or orchestra (even if the only place you play is in your garage or for your family) can not only stir your creative juices but be a way to practice Pleasure Principle #3: Connect.

Megan, Age Thirty-Six,
Adjunct Professor from Tennessee
I get my high from performing in my band, Scale
Model. I'm the singer/guitar player/lead singer. My
spirit is in absolute bliss when I'm singing and playing
with my band mates (including my husband on guitar)
in front of an audience. There's nothing better! When
I'm up on stage, I forget about all my troubles and am
totally living in the moment. The energy I feel from
the audience and the energy of playing with my band
mates, who are also in their own bliss, is better than
any drug.

There are places online where you can go to create your
own mix and mix it up with friends. Touted as a "new way
to make music with your friends," Soundstation.com acts
as an online professional music studio, with all the func-
tionality of a professional desktop digital audio worksta-
tion, including real-time effects, virtual instruments,
and recording. It's all online and accessible through your
browser. Soundstation.com has over seven hundred free
loops and samples, but you can also browse the sound shop
for more. The site also offers a premium sound library with
more than eight thousand downloadable sounds.

Once you've finished laying down your tracks, you can
share them with the world by publishing them on your own
web page, complete with a waveform player. (A waveform
player is software that makes a cloud of visual sound waves
that you can style and color.) You can also post your track
to a group for even more exposure. (Warning: Be careful
with what you post because there is no taking back what
you have floated into the cloud.)

Keys to Joy

I love to play the piano. I used to play quite a bit as a
kid, and taught for a while as an adult, but I've gotten
so busy that I don't have a ton of time to practice. This
used to cause me quite a bit of stress; I'd berate myself
for not being as dedicated of a player as I could be, but
now I've learned to just enjoy playing the few songs
that I already know and, perhaps, learn some new
ones when I have time. Don't be a perfectionist with
hobbies. It's not work, it's supposed to be fun, so being
self-critical can take away the benefits of what you like
to do in your spare time. Just enjoy!

—Beth

Lift Your Voice (and Spirits) in Song

Singing is unquestionably a way to relieve anxiety, especially
if you're singing upbeat music that puts you in a good mood
(think "Happy" by Pharrell Williams, which has recently
put smiles on people's faces). If you don't have talent like
Pharrell but want to go vocal, stick to the shower or karaoke
machine. If you're not sure whether you have a good voice,
ask someone you trust to tell you the truth. You can join a
choir (gospel or secular), a community chorus (school, local
theater, Gilbert and Sullivan troupe), or a rock or hip-hip
band. Or ask the manager of a cabaret or coffee house if you
can do a set.

**Nancy, Age Seventy-Nine,
Political Activist from California**

I go to monthly Harmony's Way meetings, where we
all get high singing a cappella. There is no songbook
or arrangements. We go around the circle, and each
person in turn starts a song, usually an old ballad
or sea shanty or gospel song—some with a chorus

or refrain that we can all join in on—and we make
up our own harmonies. There are studies about the
health benefits of singing together and about children
who sing or make music in a group becoming more
empathetic. I do it for the high and for the love of it.

Whatever your musical genre, exercising your vocal
chords will help you live a more harmonious life. Caveat:
few make it from YouTube to Madison Square Garden or
The Voice, so sing for fun rather than profit. If you happen to
make money doing it, so much the better.

If you want to let your digital diva or divo out, one online
site that allows you to create a playlist of songs is SingSnap;
it provides the lyrics to follow along while you sing. Hook
up your computer camera, if you dare, and watch yourself
(and friends) in action on your computer or TV. Again, be
careful with what you post for the world to see (I can't say
this enough). I watched someone on SingSnap dressed in
a cow suit performing in some unfamiliar tongue. It was
udderly awful!

Lorraine, Age Forty-Five,
Theater Development Fundraiser from New York
Music is a big stress reliever for me. I don't listen to
iPods because I'm always hearing music in my head.
I was a performer and singer for many years, and in
1995 I was in *Master Class* on Broadway understudying
for Audra MacDonald. It was a few days after opening
night, and I had to go on. I'd never done the show
before. The audience started roaring and applauding
when I came out for my curtain call, which was one of
the biggest highs I've ever had! I walked off stage, and
you know the expression about your knees going weak?
Well, that's what happened to me! I nearly fainted.

You don't have to be on Broadway to feel that kind of positive feedback and approval. School productions, community theater, choruses, and choirs can all give you the same kind of high. One of the first times I was on stage was in an orchestra playing cello. Hearing the full orchestral sound with the rumble of the drums sent chills up my spine—still does. Someone once said to me, "I don't know if opera is good or bad, but I can feel the hairs raise on the back of my head."

Write Now

Writing of any kind, whether it's in a journal, on a blog, or on a website like Wattpad or Figment, not only is one of the most accessible means of self-expression but also can be therapeutic. You don't have to be a professional writer to capture your most personal thoughts and emotions in a poem, a short story, or a piece of creative nonfiction. Transforming your private thoughts and feelings into a living document you can share with others can be emotionally cathartic and personally validating.

If you are interested in seriously exploring your talent as a writer, you can sign up for a creative writing course and take your work for a test drive by sharing it with others. You have to be able to take criticism if you go this route, because, as any writer knows, including this one, the only way you will get better is by editing and revising.

Kathleen, Age Sixty, from Washington

I wasn't published until after I turned forty. Now even though I work full time and have teenaged grandsons constantly draining me emotionally and financially, if I give myself time to write on my latest novel or nonfiction, I feel euphoric for hours afterwards.

If you don't have the scribe in you, reciting or memorizing poetry or lyrics that resonate is another powerful way to buoy your spirits. You can hold a salon in your house or apartment and invite guests to share a poem or passage from a book they love. Go to poets.org or songlyrics.com for inspiration. You can also go to a reading at your local bookstore or library, or to a poetry slam, which is a spoken-word competition.

Poetry Slam Dunk
In August 1988, the first poetry slam was held in New York City at the Nuyorican Poets Café, where anyone with nerves and words of steel was welcome to grab a mike and say it freestyle. In 1990, the first National Poetry Slam took place in San Francisco, with teams from Chicago and the Bay Area and one lone wolf from New York. As of 2010, the National Poetry Slam has become a word sport, currently featuring eighty certified teams each year for five days of composition—I mean competition. Slams are now held all over the world from Azerbaijan to New Zealand.

When asked about the secret to being a good writer, professionals say two things most often: Read good writing, and set aside a time to write and stick to it—put in the time, even if it's only to ramble on the page, otherwise known as "stream of consciousness." Immersing yourself in a well-written story, poem, essay, or novel can take you out of the mundane world with its cares and troubles and open your mind to new ideas and worlds like no other experience—or high. And the writers who move and impress you the most can become role models and muses that inspire your own work, whether it's for your eyes only or for possible publication. Take it from me, writing can send you—and your spirit—to new heights.

The Visual Arts

Art therapy can be beneficial to children with disabilities, people in prisons, and people who have disorders such as depression or addiction. But the truth is anyone can use the visual arts to express themselves creatively, reduce stress, or get in touch with their feelings. Remember how we freely expressed ourselves through art as children, whether it was drawing with crayons, finger painting, using watercolors, or sculpting with clay or play dough? Sadly, as adults we often lose some of our spontaneity and drive to create, and the majority of the art we do is doodles we draw during meetings or while talking on the phone. As with music, writing, or any form of self-expression, the point isn't perfection, fame, or money—it's to unleash your creative spirit and get in touch with that joy and freedom that children naturally experience if left to their own devices. The following are just a few reasons for us to get back in touch with our inner five-year-old.

Making Art to Alleviate Stress

The mere act of drawing and creating art can help us alleviate stress in several ways.

Distraction. So you had a tiff with a colleague at work, or you fought with your spouse. Get out a sketch pad, and draw something to take your mind off of what's making you anxious—even if it's just for a few minutes. When you are finished being engrossed in your sketches, you'll have a clearer head with which to tackle your problems.

Flow. Experts say art creates a quality called flow, which refers to being engaged in something that puts you in a meditative state, where your mind is cleared of interfering thoughts. This artful flow has much of the same benefits of meditation, leaving you feeling more relaxed when you are done.

Self-care. Having a creative outlet, such as making art, can make you feel more balanced in your life, especially if you are dragged down by the worries of work, parenting, elder care, financial stress, illness, or other issues. With all of our responsibilities, we often forget that we need and deserve time to take care of ourselves. By taking time to create art, even if it's for a short period, you not only will rejuvenate your spirit but will have something beautiful (or at least a conversation piece) to show for it!

DIY Art Therapy

One of the best DIY stress relievers for budding artists is keeping a sketchbook (the art equivalent to a writing journal). Keeping a sketchbook can be cathartic, creative, and anxiety-reducing. Here are a few ideas for using a sketchbook for stress management:

- Draw something that represents how you are feeling about what's happening in your life and the things that are causing you stress. This exercise can be a way of processing your emotions. (I experimented with this during a particularly anxious period and drew a rendering of Edvard Munch's *The Scream*. If you're not familiar with this painting, you can look it up online.)

- Sketch pictures that express your feelings about a stressful event from the past. Many have found this experience to be healing. Note: If you are severely anxious or depressed, you might want to discuss your images and the feelings they evoke with a therapist or psychologist.

- Keep a dream sketch diary. Draw scenes from dreams you'd like to remember or better understand. (Again, you can discuss these with a professional, if you wish.)

- Keep a beauty sketch diary. Draw the faces of those you love, places you find peaceful, or flowers and landscapes you think are lovely. Looking back at drawings of things that you find beautiful is a way of revisiting happier times, especially during periods of stress (Photos also work to jog pleasant memories.) You can also just make art a part of your everyday life, stress or no stress.

- Visit a museum or gallery, and sit quietly gazing at a beautiful landscape or portrait. Impressionist paintings do it for me, but whatever style of art you enjoy can rejuvenate your spirit and evoke pleasant thoughts. Steer clear of surrealist paintings if you're feeling on edge. If you aren't, surrealists and other painters, such as Hieronymus Bosch and René Magritte, can be pretty trippy, if that's your kind of high. On the other end of the spectrum are the landscape painters, who can both soothe and stir you with their dramatic scenes of natural beauty.

- The website drawsketch.about.com is devoted to drawing and sketching for people of all skill levels. It offers a newsletter and free stress management classes to boot.

- You can also sign up for art classes at your local community college, YMCA, YWCA, or JCC (Jewish Community Center).

So get out your sketch pad, finger paints, crayons, and brushes, and have some fun!

The Art of Hobbies and Crafts

The so-called fine arts aren't the only way to be creative and express your inner spirit. Hobbies such as gardening, cooking, and scrapbooking as well as traditional crafts like woodworking, crocheting, quilt-making (a good activity for socializing), making pottery, and sewing—the list goes on— require great creativity and can be the vehicles for personal expression that have the same effect on stress and the brain as meditation, music, and painting.

Create Your Garden of Eden

Find a place and create your own garden. Planting new things which are unique can help release some of your pent-up stress. Gardening is not just being with nature—it's creating it!

—Zeda

Note: Live in a city? Transform your roof or terrace into a garden, or join a garden group in your local park.

Pot Lucky

Why not make cooking a hobby? Most people dread coming home from work and making dinner. Scour cookbooks and the Internet for new recipes; make your grocery shopping trip an adventure by buying ingredients that are new to you. Turn on some music, and make cooking fun! It can be a great stress reliever, plus, it's something you have to do anyway. Try some dishes you haven't had before to widen your horizons.

—Dayiannaki

Note: Trying out new recipes and food is good for your brain by producing new neural connections—not to mention human ones;

people are more than happy to sit down at your table for some home-cooked meals.

Darn It

I'm not very good at crocheting, but there is one thing I make regularly—scarves. I love doing it! Being able to crochet basic things gives me something to do if I want to just get into a meditative state, and it also allows me to join knitting circles and yarn clubs, where I can connect with my friends who are much more creative than I am in this hobby, without having to put too much time into it.

—The Crochet Queen

Note: The Crochet Queen rules by combining two Pleasure Principles—creating and socializing.

So You Think You Can Dance?

Do you have the moves like Mick Jagger or Beyoncé? Or is shifting from one foot to the other your idea of busting a move? Whatever the case, when you're feeling tense, you might want to turn up the tunes and shake your booty—or put on some Tchaikovsky and leap around your living room with abandon! I've been dancing since I was a little girl in tap shoes and a tutu, and it still does wonders for me. Here's why.

The 2008 documentary *Gotta Dance* is anecdotal proof that dancing can keep us young. In it, director Dori Berinstein chronicled the debut of the New Jersey Nets' first ever senior hip-hop dance team, the NJ NETSationals. This group of twelve women and one man, then ages sixty to eighty-one, made headlines after being chosen as cheerleaders after an audition. This delightful film shows how these inspirational, ordinary folks transformed their lives by learning dance steps and wowing the fans with their dare-to-break-hip-hop moves.

Not only is dancing fun and creative, it also instills grace, supports good posture, and boosts your brain power. According to a study in the *New England Journal of Medicine*, dancing can improve your memory and, in some cases, slow down or prevent the development of dementia as you get older.

Donna Flagg, Age Forty-Nine,
Dance and Movement Teacher from New York
I feel high when I dance, and after I'm done I feel even higher. When I was a kid, I would stay home from school with a 104 degree fever, but still go to dance class for three or four hours, feel terrific, and then collapse afterwards. It is my go-to drug, and it has helped me heal from awful breakups, grieve through the sadness of deaths, and even lifted me up from the grind of just the everyday restrictive feelings of life. Dancing has been the greatest gift of joy and healing in my life. As a dancer and teacher I get to share this gift of integration between body, self, and mind, to others.

Even if all you can muster is jumping up and down rave-style (great exercise, by the way) or following the person next to you in a line dance, it's all good. The truth is that no one is looking at you unless you're auditioning. Most people are too concerned about whether *they* look foolish, so being self-conscious on the dance floor wastes precious time and energy. And if you want to get the full benefits of dancing, you must *feel* the music, which comes from the inside. This can be a transformative experience if you let yourself go with the flow.

The same goes for painting, writing, or playing an instrument. So what if your violin squeaks or your clarinet honks like a Canada goose?

Clark, Age Fifty, Teacher from California
My wife and I invited friends to our house ceilidh, a Celtic tradition where people would gather together to play folk music or dance. We asked guests to bring something to share: poems, songs, short stories, music, even juggling—whatever they wanted to perform. Afterwards, we all danced the ceilidh, which is what the social gathering is named after. We all had a blast, and it was fantastic seeing how talented our friends are!

While it's true many people are naturally gifted in many of the arts, which is why we have museums and concert halls, this shouldn't stop you from pursuing any or all of these ways to practice this Pleasure Principle. Use it to express and expand your inner self. Art is a celebration of our creative spirit, one of the many ways we celebrate life, the subject of the next chapter.

Pleasure Principle #5

Celebrate

Affirming Life, Experiencing Joy

Laughter is wine for the soul—laughter soft, or loud and deep,
tinged through with seriousness the hilarious declaration
made by man that life is worth living.

—Seán O'Casey, Irish dramatist

Celebrations, as you read earlier in the chapter on the history of getting high, have always been one of our favorite and most pleasurable pastimes. Whether it's a birthday, wedding, graduation, christening, Bar or Bat Mitzvah, anniversary, Halloween, Valentine's Day, Fourth of July, Memorial Day, Labor Day, or religious holidays from Christmas to Ramadan, people love gathering together with friends and family to celebrate with food, gifts, dancing, singing, and some fun and frivolity. And while many also mark these milestones and holidays with mood-altering substances, you don't have to drink or use chemicals to experience the high spirits of any occasion. These are occasions to celebrate your family, friends, and community that are your Connecting Circles from Pleasure Principle #3 and to affirm the joy—the high—of simply being alive.

Laughter Really
Is the Best Medicine

You have probably heard that it takes more muscles to frown than to smile, which is factually correct. Also true, according to a Michigan State University study, is that smiling can alleviate the pain of an upsetting situation and improve your mood. Chuckling has been shown to help people perform better on cognitive tasks.

In another university study, humor associated with mirthful laughter (HAML) was found to be a viable non-pharmacological practice that promotes greater wholeness, health, and wellness. HAML was also shown to help alleviate symptoms from a variety of chronic medical conditions.

"What we have found is that humor actually engages the entire brain," explained Lee Berk, principal investigator of the study and associate professor at the School of Allied Health Professions at Loma Linda University. "It is a whole brain experience with a gamma wave band frequency similar to meditation. This is of great value to individuals who need or want to revisit, reorganize, or rearrange various aspects of their lives or experiences to make them feel whole or more focused Laughter isn't only good medicine for the health of your body but also a good medicine for your brain."

And a way to celebrate the joy of living, I might add.

**Natalie, Age Twenty-Nine,
Bookkeeper from California**
I was feeling depressed so I decided to sign up for Laughing Yoga. Even though it's called yoga, there are no positions or meditation involved. It consisted of theater game exercises where participants act out scenarios. One time we pretended to be talking on the phone with someone on the other end who is saying something hilarious. There was a lot of "ho, ho, ho-ing"

in nonspontaneous laughter. Most of the time we would stand in a circle and the leader would say various things and ask us to laugh at the end of them.

"And we are the greatest!" the leader would shout, followed by call-and-response laughing. Everyone took a few steps towards the center of the group, raised their hands up in the air, and chuckled. There were also partner exercises. It was hard not to feel foolish sometimes, but overcoming that feeling is part of the method. Laughing Yoga helped lift my mood when I was going through a hard time. This technique is now being offered at the University of California, San Francisco, so it's becoming more respected and popular.

Laughter as Therapy

Ten years ago, Dr. Madan Kataria burst out laughing for no reason at all. Since then he's helped form over three thousand Laughter Clubs throughout India, working toward the goal of creating a million such clubs around the world. In India, Laughter Clubs are now commonplace, and members meet outside on a daily basis in public parks or community centers.

Dan Nainan, Age Fifty-Three, Comedian from New York

I never drank, smoked, or did drugs, so the only highs I know about are natural. I truly believe there are no feelings that you can get when you're high that you can't get without drugs. Before I became a comedian I saw a lot of stand-up comedy. I love to laugh and to make people laugh. The ability to tell a joke that I might have thought of in the shower and make a roomful of people crack up is the greatest high in the world. There are actually laughing clubs

in India where people get together to laugh for five to
ten minutes in the mornings before going to work. It's
extremely therapeutic and a great way to start the day.
The only problem is, if this catches on here in the US,
it could put us comedians out of business! If you think
about it, it doesn't matter what language you speak or
what culture you are from, laughter sounds the same
all over the world. That says something about the
universal power of laughter.

"When you laugh, you change," explains Kataria, whose
fans include actors Goldie Hawn and John Cleese. "And
when you change, the whole world changes around you."
Shouldn't he have said, "When you laugh, the world laughs
with you"?

Why Laughter Therapy Works

Laughter Therapy can be done by anyone at any age. You
can do laughing exercises in the privacy of your home,
but it's recommended that you laugh with others, as it is
a great social and bonding experience, and it's contagious
(in a good way). Laughing in a group will encourage you to
lose your inhibitions. With Laughter Therapy, whether in
a Laughter Club or in the comfort of your home, the exercises are simple to follow, and they don't require any special
clothes or equipment.

Laughing exercises the abdominal muscles, the joints,
the spine, the diaphragm, and the muscles of the face. You
take in four to six times as much oxygen while laughing
than when you are sedentary and do not laugh. Your heart
rate increases, and your blood flows faster through the
arteries. Chemical neurotransmitters produce pain-killing
and tranquilizing endorphins in the brain. Laughing even
burns calories!

Vacation as Celebration

August marks the official beginning of summer vacation for Europe, which, unlike the United States, believes time off is a right not a luxury. Ironically, the month when many Americans take their two-week break—if they're lucky enough to have accrued that much time off or are not on that extended holiday otherwise known as unemployment—is the same time when finding an actual European in their native country is like a game of Where's Waldo?

Even economic downturns are not enough to keep the continentals from enjoying their downtime. According to a report by the Center for Economic and Policy Research, European countries lead the world in guaranteeing paid leave for their workers. Spain and Germany are among the most holiday-happy, both offering thirty-four days of paid leave each year. Italy and France guarantee thirty-one days of paid vacation, and Belgium has thirty. These numbers include both mandatory vacation and public holidays. New Zealand and Australia guarantee thirty and twenty-eight days of paid leave respectively, and Canada's federal government stipulates nineteen paid days, with some provinces adding on additional time. On the opposite end of the spectrum is Japan, where thousands commit suicide every year because of work-related stress: all workers are guaranteed ten paid vacation days.

I recall one Australian I met while traveling through Europe in my early twenties who asked me how long I was on vacation. When I told him two weeks, thinking that was a generous amount of time to take off in one chunk, he stared at me with pity. "That's it!?" he said incredulously. "I'm on holiday for two months."

Nowadays, few American employees take two weeks' vacation at once, preferring to add days to national holidays in order to extend their time off, or maybe take Fridays during the summer to get long weekends. But, according to one source, the average vacation for most people is just four days; when you factor in travel time, that's about twenty-four hours of real R&R. Because many people quit or get laid off before they've accrued vacation days, few people really get the chance to enjoy their time off. A two-month vacation, like the one my Aussie friend took, is for those on maternity leave or disability.

Lest you think these other countries are a bunch of slackers, think again. Studies show Americans have a lot to learn about avoiding burnout and that vacations are good for both our mental health and the health of our economy.

The sad fact is that Americans are vacation-deprived. The United States is the only advanced nation that does not provide a legal guarantee of paid leave. And even when they are given vacation time, Americans often choose to stay put. The average American worker was given fourteen days of vacation during the past year, for example, yet took only ten, leaving four days unused, twice as many as the previous year. Collectively, Americans failed to take an estimated 577,212,000 available days of vacation, according to a 2013 Vacation Deprivation survey by Expedia, an online travel company.

The weak economy makes some people never leave their workplace out of fear that they will be blamed for something that goes awry while they are away, or that their boss will suddenly realize that they are expendable. Add the stress of planning, travel expenses (gas or airline fees), and finding a kennel for your dog, should you have one, and you have an overworked workforce. Still, here are some undisputed truths about taking time off:

- *A relaxed employee is a more productive employee.*
  Stressed-out workers make more mistakes than
  well-rested ones.

- *Vacations promote creativity.* A good vacation can help us reconnect with ourselves and our loved ones. It gives us a fresh perspective on our lives and promotes introspection and positive self-discovery, all of which helps us feel our best.

- *Vacations prevent burnout.* Workers who take regular time to relax are less likely to experience burnout and tend to enjoy their jobs more than those who never take a break.

- *Vacations can keep us healthier and happier.* Taking regular time off to recharge your batteries, thereby keeping stress levels lower, can keep you healthier. One study found that three days after a vacation, subjects' physical complaints, quality of sleep, and mood had improved compared to before the vacation. These gains lasted a full five weeks, especially in those who had a good time during their vacations.

- *Vacations can strengthen bonds.* Spending time enjoying life with loved ones can keep relationships strong, helping you enjoy the good times more and manage the stress of the hard times. In fact, a study by the Arizona Department of Health and Human Services found that women who took vacations were more satisfied with their marriages. Listen up, spouses. Happy wife, happy life!

The bottom line is to give yourself a break if you want to reduce the stress in your life. As the well-known adage goes, no one on their deathbed has ever said they wished they had spent more time at work. Of course, not everyone can afford to take a vacation, especially an extended one (unless you're European, of course). For those who just can't get away, here are some staycation ideas.

Add an extra day to your weekend, even if you just stay at home in your PJs and read a stack of magazines or books. (Tip: don't answer the phone or check your email.) Or you might want to take a personal day from work and go to a movie during the day, especially one that you want to see and maybe your spouse or partner does not. Enjoy your leisure time sitting in the darkness of a nearly empty theater with surround sound in one of those comfy reclining seats that many theaters now have.

Book a night or two at a hotel or B&B in or near where you live, and it can feel like a holiday or a romantic getaway. Make sure you don't eat out at one of your regular haunts (no matter how much you love it). Go to a new restaurant, or try a different type of cuisine.

Drive or take the train to a town or city that you've never been to, and explore the restaurants, shops, and local events. A few hours in any direction can feel like a cultural exploration. One New York City family I know took out a subway map and had their kids point to a station stop where they would all go visit for a day. That and the train fare will get you a cheap diversion.

Be a tourist in your own town. You'd be surprised what you *don't* know about where you live. As someone who spent nearly an entire summer at my desk writing this book, I finally looked out my window at the passing Circle Line (a cruise ship for tourists) sailing along the Hudson, got myself a ticket, and rode the waves. I learned about where they filmed the movie *On the Waterfront* (New Jersey, who knew?) and about the site of the since-demolished Domino Sugar Factory that once sweetened New York City's coastline. Afterwards I wrote a review about my experience for Travelocity called "Circle of Swell" for what is now a regular "Tourist in My Own City" series. The Empire State Building is next. I haven't been to the observation deck in years, but

I've seen it in enough films (*Sleepless in Seattle, King Kong,* and *An Affair to Remember* to name just 3 out of 250.)

Have a spa day. My husband's idea of bliss involves the ocean, sand, and a run along the beach, but this sun-sensitive hermit crab would rather take a dip in a whirlpool and get a massage, mani-pedi, and facial. It's my idea of heaven on earth (and I'm not alone in this). Look online for coupons and specials, or do a discount search. There's nothing like feeling the stress melt away while wrapped in a terry cloth bathrobe and wearing floppy slippers.

Make a play date. Remember how those fun-loving Puritans got relief from their daily drudgery by playing games with their families? You might need to stop Candy Crushing (or whatever game app you're addicted to) and play some old-school games like chess, checkers, Clue, Monopoly, Pictionary, Trivial Pursuit, Password, Life, and Risk and have a family game night. There's a reason these games have lasted for generations. Kinect or Wii is okay, too, if it involves more than one player, but there is something special about live group games of strategy that seem to last forever and are fun as well as intellectually challenging.

Go on a picnic. When's the last time you packed up a basket of goodies and a blanket to have an outdoor lunch with your family, friends, or partner? Take turns telling your favorite joke or anecdote. You can roast marshmallows at the park or on the beach (I recommend dusk—a good time to tell ghost stories). Don't forget to use all your senses to take in the sights and sounds around you. Take deep breaths of fresh air, and allow for some quiet time to listen to the wind rustling through the leaves or the crash of waves against the shore. (You are combining several Pleasure Principles here— having fun, connecting with nature, and socializing.) Make sure to clean up your mess when you're done, and be careful to douse the flame completely before you leave. (I am an environmental evangelist, and nothing irks me more than seeing someone else's debris carelessly left behind.)

Gratitude

If we don't feel grateful for what we already have,
what makes us think we'd be happy with more?

—Unknown author

Celebrating life starts with being grateful. If you don't feel gratitude, you cannot experience true pleasure, because without it you are just going through the motions. The act of living in gratitude is the shield that protects us from our day-to-day struggles and pain. Why is gratitude so important? Because if you are grateful for all you have and all you've been given, it is difficult to encounter an obstacle you cannot deal with. Gratitude is what keeps us from falling into a pit of despair when bad stuff happens to us.

Try this exercise: At the end of the day, write down one or more things that you are grateful for or something that happened to you that day for which you would like to give thanks. It's okay to repeat from day to day. You can include people on your list as well. If you are so inclined, you can write a thank-you note or email to those people to let them know how much you appreciate them. Writing thank-you notes is a lost art, but there is no one who doesn't enjoy getting one.

Keeping a gratitude journal is good for children so they don't take the gifts that life or loving parents give them for granted. It acts as a human spoiler alert. Our family plays a game called Traffic Light at the dinner table. Red is the bad stuff that happened that day, green is the good, and yellow is for what we have to look forward to. It's another fun way to assess our day and to count our blessings.

Keep it simple. You can be grateful for a good night's sleep or for your friend or sibling who listened to your latest rant and gave you some good advice or comfort. Once you start becoming aware of the little gifts that come your way every day, you will find that your list will expand, and you will notice more and more of life's everyday miracles. I'm not saying that you will always have a good day, but noticing the good things that happen will help offset the negative things.

Glennon Doyle Melton is the author of a terrific book called *Carry On, Warrior.* On her Momastery blog she writes:

> Recently I posted a picture of myself in my kitchen, and I immediately started receiving generous messages from people wanting to help me "update" it. Along with their messages came pictures of how my kitchen could look, if I'd just put some effort and money into it. I've always loved my kitchen, but after seeing those pictures I found myself looking at it through new, critical eyes. Maybe it *was* all wrong. Maybe the 80's counters, laminate cabinets, mismatched appliances and clutter really *were* mistakes I should try to fix. I stood and stared and suddenly my kitchen looked shabby and lazy to me. I wondered if that meant I was shabby and lazy, too. Because our kitchens are nothing if not reflections of us, right?
>
> But as I lay down to sleep, I remembered this passage from Thoreau's *Walden*: "I say beware of all enterprises that require new clothes and not a new wearer of the clothes." *Walden* reminds me that when I feel lacking, I don't need new things, I need new eyes with which to see the things I already have.

So when I woke up this morning, I walked into my kitchen wearing fresh perspectacles. Here's what I saw.

You guys. I have a REFRIGERATOR.

This thing MAGICALLY MAKES FOOD COLD. I'm pretty sure in the olden days, frontierswomen had to drink warm Diet Coke. Sweet Jesus. Thank you, precious kitchen.

Inside my refrigerator is FOOD. Healthy food that so many parents would give anything to be able to feed their children. Almost 16,000 mama's babies die every day from malnutrition. Not mine. When this food runs out, I'll just jump in my car to get more. It's ludicrous, really. It's like my family hits the lottery every freaking morning.

And for this post, I say, thank you, Glennon. Thank you for getting it! Now go give thanks to your fridge, coffeemaker, and dishwasher if you are lucky enough to have one. My circa-1890 apartment doesn't. Not that I'm complaining (well, maybe a little bit), but thanks for the washing machine in the basement, even if I have to feed it money to make it run. At least I'm not using a washboard by the river.

Celebrating Milestones Can Improve Relationships

Most couples remember the landmark moments in their relationship: the first time they met, the day they were engaged, their wedding, the birth of their children. But as time goes by and familiarity breeds, if not contempt, flagging interest, marking these special occasions often falls to the wayside or gets dropped from the list of priorities.

Research shows, however, that celebrating important milestones in one's life can actually help strengthen relationships. If you are having problems as a couple, taking the time to celebrate together will bring back memories of those happier times. Talking about the good memories, including the romantic dates and fun vacations (yes, vacations) will remind you why you fell in love in the first place and help you focus on the good qualities in your relationship rather than the annoying way he chews with his mouth open. (Can you tell I've been married for a while?)

Celebrations also create new memories. Good relationships are built on pleasurable memories, and without them couples can find themselves sitting across from one another at the dinner table in silence, especially when the kids are not the focal point of the discussion because they are either out of the house or busy with their own pleasure seeking.

Look at old photographs to help spark a conversation about something fun you did together in the past. Then plan to recreate that day. It doesn't have to be a huge event—even spending a weekend together doing something out of the ordinary, or going out to a romantic dinner to talk about the fact that you are still a team after all these years, can be a way to celebrate.

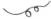

All the family and friend milestones—birthdays, graduations, holidays, weddings, even funerals—can be a celebration of relationships and a reminder to be grateful for the support and joy the people in your life bring. These are also times to give back in return for what they've given you: expressions of your love and gratitude that will strengthen your bonds with your friends and loved ones for years to come.

Which takes us to Pleasure Principle #6: Give.

Pleasure Principle #6

Give

Being of Service, Finding Purpose

Carry out a random act of kindness, with no expectation
of reward, safe in the knowledge that one day
someone might do the same for you.

—Princess Diana

Countless religions teach us that helping others is not only a worthy pursuit but a moral obligation. But donating either your time (the best) or your money (also great, especially if given willingly and not just as a tax break) is like a boomerang of positivity. Science now tells us that charity work is good for our mind, body, and spirit. A recent study by the University of North Carolina found that the type of happiness that comes from helping others and having a larger purpose in life produces more antibodies than other types of pleasurable pursuits, which helps us ward off illnesses. In addition to making us happier, the social interaction that volunteering entails can lower your heart rate and blood pressure, increase endorphin production, enhance your immune system, and shield you against stress.

Noted spiritual teacher and author Deepak Chopra says we should not think of service in the conventional sense, as in one's duty, but to look at it from the perspective of higher states of consciousness. In this view, service is not only a humanitarian effort but a path of joy and self-realization (our highest sense of self and purpose). It is an opportunity to increase our happiness. Service is about acting on a call for the unique gifts we can offer others. When this is a genuine calling, it isn't based on our ego needs or motivated by social expectations.

People in recovery from addiction who work a Twelve Step program learn that service is key to staying clean and sober. Using alcohol or other drugs can make us feel isolated from the rest of the world (especially from those who do not use). Addicts, by their obsession with using, tend to be narcissistic, thinking only about their own immediate needs and neglecting those around them, including family and friends. By being a sponsor or reaching out to newcomers in their AA or NA groups, recovering alcoholics and addicts give back and keep their own demons at bay while helping others stay sober.

It might be hard to believe if you are caught up in your own misery, but there is someone out there who is in more pain than you are now and is in need of help. Just turn on or read the news, and you will find millions of people who are suffering from war, poverty, and natural or unnatural disasters.

Aside from the overwhelmingly positive feeling you get from giving unselfishly to others, you are likely to meet new people whose values you can admire and emulate. Being of service to others is a way to take you out of your own head for a while and forget your own troubles.

The act of compassion validates us in a profound way and creates a deep connection that heals by overcoming that feeling of isolation. When we offer compassion to others, something happens to us spiritually—our happiness and sense of well-being grow exponentially.

Paying It Forward

As Mukta Khalsa, director of the Kripalu Center for Yoga and Health in New Mexico, told me in a phone interview: "Life is about what we can do for others. It's not just about me, me, me, but about the greater We. Ask yourself, 'How else can I serve humanity?' Giving and sharing creates an elevation of consciousness, which is a natural high."

Here are just three of the benefits of paying it forward.

Giving increases self-confidence and self-esteem. Evidence suggests that helping others can lead to a sense of greater self-worth and confidence, and volunteering can provide you with a sense of purpose, especially during tough times.

Giving encourages friendships that buffer us against stress. Volunteering gives you the opportunity to meet and connect with new people. It helps widen your social networks, which we know can stave off the depression that comes with feeling lonely.

Volunteering might help you live longer. Studies show evidence that being actively involved in ongoing volunteer work can increase your life expectancy, while improving your quality of life. And the earlier you start the better. Research tells us that people who volunteer when they are younger experience better health outcomes later on in life. So if you have been thinking about joining a charity, read on to discover the myriad possibilities and carpe diem (seize the day)!

To find a charity in your area, go to volunteer.org, or explore some of the following good causes.

Become a Big Sister or Big Brother. Become a mentor to an underprivileged child, age six to eighteen, who doesn't have a grown-up to look up to. Go to a ballgame, play in the park, take a walk in the woods, or help a teen get a job or internship. The relationships and the memories you will make with these kids can last a lifetime, and you will have the opportunity to indelibly change a life. Go to bbbs.org.

Work at your local food bank. Times are tough, and many people are going hungry these days. If you have the means and the time, roll up your sleeves, and pack some breakfast, lunchboxes, and dinners for the one in six Americans who are food insecure. See feedingamerica.org/find-your-local-foodbank/.

Sign up for a charity walk. Nearly every disease or charity has a walk, run, or bike ride to raise money for research to find a cure. It's usually only one day a year, and because it involves some form of exercise, it combines two Pleasure Principles and doesn't require much of your time. Check your local papers, blogs, and social service organizations for lists of upcoming events.

The Right Path

In their newest book, *A Path Appears*, Pulitzer-winning husband-and-wife team Nicholas Kristof and Sheryl WuDunn wrote about how each of us can best give and the lasting benefits we gain in return. As they state in their introduction:

> A generation ago, we didn't have much more than hunches to guide us in trying to make a difference and build a life of greater meaning and satisfaction. "Giving back" was then what we did in December, hunched over a checkbook and relying on guesswork. In recent years . . . advances in neuroscience and economics—and a flowering of carefully monitored experiments—have given us much greater insight into what works to create oppor-

tunity worldwide, and much greater prospects for personal satisfaction from giving. That's partly why we chose our title from an essay by the great Chinese writer Lu Xun. A path is now appearing to show us how to have a positive impact on the world around us. This is a path of hopefulness, but also a path of fulfillment: typically, we start off by trying to empower others and end up empowering ourselves, too.

As Kristof and WuDunn acknowledge in their beautiful book, giving is something that most of us *want* to do, but many don't because we end up stuck in the muddy ditch of complacency. Maybe we feel we don't have the time, or, like Scarlet O'Hara in *Gone with the Wind*, we tell ourselves that there's always tomorrow. Unfortunately, life has a way of whizzing by, and when misfortune or illness strikes, we are suddenly the one in need of a helping hand. If you feel you want to help but don't know what to do, VolunteerMatch .org or Idealist.org is a good start. You can and should check out the credentials of charitable organizations by going to Charity Navigator, CharityWatch, Philanthropedia, or the Better Business Bureau's Wise Giving Alliance. (This is especially recommended if you plan to make a financial gift.)

Below are some examples of worthy causes that have already been vetted by charity watchdogs. They range from helping veterans, the poor, and animals in need, to finding a cure for cancer.

The Humane Society

The Humane Society of the United States [humane society.org] create[s] a humane and sustainable world for all animals, including people, through education, advocacy, and the promotion of respect and compassion.

**Diane, Age Fifty-Five, Publicist
and Animal Shelter Volunteer from New York**
I got into helping animals after I ended a relationship and I was feeling lost. I thought animal shelter volunteering would achieve two goals: doing something I was passionate about, which has always been animals, and possibly making new friends. Since volunteering and now working for pay at an animal shelter, I have realized both these goals. All these years I've worked with celebrities as a publicist, and there is a kind of rush I got when my clients got on the national TV shows or lots of press, and I felt that I did my job successfully.

But when I'm adopting out the animals, I get a different and better kind of rush. People will come up to me at the shelter and say, "God bless you for what you do." The first few times I heard that, I didn't think much of it. Now I never get tired of hearing that. When I see an animal that is shut down because it had a horrible life or came from a puppy mill, and I'm able to place it in a home and get a picture from a family with the dog on the sofa or playing with a kid, I get such an amazing feeling! I feel like I'm saving lives by giving these animals a second chance. If I never see another drug again for the rest of my life, I'd be thrilled. Animal rescue is the most incredible high I ever could have.

The International Cancer Advocacy Network (ICAN)
ICAN [askican.org] provides Personalized Medicine Cancer Case Management Programs, through its customized patient advocacy services to Stage IV

patients who have been written off by their oncology teams. The organization specializes in complex and rare diagnoses, whether pediatric or adult cancers. ICAN, given years of experience with oncology issues and the anticancer drug pipeline, assists patients in the battle to extend life with high quality of life through physician referrals, cutting-edge information and advocacy services, clinical trials research, compassionate use analysis, and palliative care program services.

Meals On Wheels

The Meals On Wheels Association of America [mow aa.org] is the oldest and largest membership organization supporting the national network of more than five thousand Senior Nutrition Programs that operate in all fifty states and the US territories. The tireless work of these programs—supported by a dedicated army of two million volunteers—delivers a nutritious meal, a warm smile, and a safety check that helps keep 2.5 million seniors healthy, safe, and living independently in their own homes each year.

Veterans of Foreign Wars National Home for Children

The VFW National Home for Children [vfwtnational home.org] helps military and veteran families find stability and positive change during times of crisis.

The Nature Generation

The Nature Generation [natgen.org], formerly the Newton Marasco Foundation, is a public environmental charity that inspires and empowers youth to make a difference. [They] reach our nation's

youth through innovative environmental steward-
ship programs in literature, science and the arts.
The Nature Generation has invested in our next
generation through Teach Green Programs and
Read Green. NatGen has reached out to thousands
of kids in 2013.

The National Association of Injured
& Disabled Workers (NAIDW)

The NAIDW [naidw.org] is a nationally recognized
non-profit educational and humanitarian organization founded on first hand life experiences
and dedicated to improving the quality of life of
injured and disabled workers and their families by
providing unlimited resources, support, guidance
and grant-based financial aid to injured and disabled workers and their families suffering from the
results of injury, illness, pain or disability! Motto:
"No worker left behind!"

Amnesty International

Amnesty International [amnesty.org] is a global
movement of more than 7 million people who campaign for a world where human rights are enjoyed
by all. We reach almost every country in the world
and have:

- more than 2 million members and
  supporters who drive forward our
  fight for rights
- more than 5 million activists who
  strengthen our calls for justice

Our vision is for every person to enjoy all the rights
enshrined in the Universal Declaration of Human

Rights and other international human rights standards.

We are independent of any government, political ideology, economic interest or religion, and are funded mainly by our membership and public donations.

Bill and Melinda Gates Foundation

The famous tech entrepreneur and his wife are devoting their time and considerable resources for global health, global development, and education initiatives that will improve the quality of life for people around the world. See the website gatesfoundation.org for more information.

Experience Corps

Run by the American Association for Retired Persons (AARP), Experience Corps (aarp.org/experience-corps) engages older adults as reading tutors for struggling students in public schools. A $100 donation can help provide books and supplies for volunteers to use in the classroom throughout the school year, or you can volunteer your services at a school near you.

For more information on where and how to volunteer, visit Network for Good's web page about volunteer opportunities: networkforgood.org/volunteer.

These are just a few selections from hundreds of organizations that need your help. Find what causes speak to your heart—that feed your sense of purpose in life—and offer your services. You will become a part of something greater than yourself, which is the definition of an expanded consciousness—of HIGH.

Hope, Forty-Eight, Volunteer High School Scholarship Chair, PTA, from Virginia

Volunteering is not all about benefiting the people you know best, but it's about helping complete strangers. The economy is discouraging students from pursuing a higher education, so I believe it's my obligation to lift some financial stress off of at least one family. I have a daughter who will go off to college in two years, and I can empathize with those parents who want to send their child off to college but just can't afford it. What do they tell their children? I know I can't help every student, but it's rewarding to have an impact on even one student's life. Volunteering not only makes a difference in the community, but it changed my perspective about what is important in life. It reminded me that the world is much bigger than just me and my family. I encourage everyone to find something that you are passionate about and become involved in it.

Of all the people who contributed to my understanding of what it means to give, no one summed up the pleasure of service more eloquently than a teenager from Montana named Nadia. She demonstrates why love is an unbreakable "chain of giving," and how making others happy will make you a happier person.

Nadia Ben-Yousseff, Age Thirteen, from Montana

I've been singing and performing poetry since I was six years old. I guess I've volunteered since I was eight. My singing is a cappella; I don't sing with music. I used to sing for my mother's friends, and then I started singing for fundraisers put on by church groups, women's clubs, and stuff like that. I have three books of poetry and songs. I donate all of the money from the books to children's charities. Money from my first book went to a school for deaf and blind kids in Great Falls, Montana, and to the Lions Club. They did a campaign called Sight First to help the blind. Money from the second book went to Home on the Range, a shelter for abused children and to the Feed the Children fund for orphans in Bosnia. I also visit people at a local nursing home. I do the women's hair, I do their nails, and they ask me to come by on Sundays and perform for them. I also sing for homebound hospice patients. I guess that's what's really fulfilling to me, when I sing to someone who is dying, someone who is really sick, and who isn't aware of much of what's happening, but when I'm done there's a smile on that person's face. I find that everyone needs love, everyone can give love. Making someone happy makes you happy, and they go on and make others happy and it's like a chain. Love is a chain of giving. You change when you get older, but love is ageless. Love is the same when you are 7, 13, or 102.

Can there be a greater high than this?

Postscript

To all of you who want more guilt-free pleasure in your lives (and who doesn't?), I suggest the following exercise: Make a list of your most memorable natural highs. They can be times when you felt elation, physical pleasure, spiritual transformation, or inner peace. Chances are they will fall into at least one of the six Pleasure Principles you just read about. I asked myself the same question and came up with many wonderful experiences, all of which were far better than anything I ever felt when chemically high.

While giving birth to a baby is a painful labor of love, there are countless moments of sheer delight that come with having children. Watching those first tentative steps, the hugs, the giggles, the family games and outings, the pride of a scored goal or hard-earned A's on a report card. Pleasure. Of course, you don't have to have children to get a natural high—there's all that care-free, child-free time to spend with your partner or with friends. And there are our other babies—every beloved pet we've ever brought into our homes.

I remember that first exciting kiss with my then-boyfriend, now my husband of many years. There was that freshly baked chocolate croissant we had for breakfast on a wind-swept beach, the fiery sun descending below the horizon in Greece, celebrating a birthday with friends on a rooftop at dusk as Manhattan's skyline shimmered in the distance, being drenched by the swells while white-water rafting, parasailing high above the cliffs of Mexico, snorkeling in the coral reefs of Key Largo, kayaking past harbor seals in Maine, gazing in awe at the vast mountain ranges of Wyoming and Colorado, the waterfalls and volcanoes of Hawaii, the view of the Golden Gate Bridge in San Francisco, and driving along California's Pacific Coast Highway. Pleasure.

There are beautifully plated and expertly prepared meals at fine restaurants way above my means and less elegant but equally delicious home-cooked meals made with love. There is dancing to one of my favorite songs at a wedding, a club, or at home, no matter how cheesy the tunes; the cleansing breaths I take while meditating or at yoga; the healing, stress-melting massages; laughing with an audience of strangers at a movie and the feeling of connection that comes with getting the same joke at the same time; a painting, play, or song executed so magnificently that my eyes well up with tears. Pleasure.

This is only a partial list of my personal highs. Now read over yours, and let your brain's reward system recall how you felt on those remarkable days and in those special moments. Then—and this is key—make a plan to recreate some of those experiences. Equally important, decide to make new memories that get you just as high. It might be helpful to make another wish list and include the most positive people in your life so you can get together with them.

Joy is contagious. Pass it on, and don't forget to pay it forward.

References

Chapter 1: Doing It Old School

Al-Qur'an: A Contemporary Translation by Ahmed Ali. Princeton, NJ: Princeton University Press, 1984.

"Ancient Olympic Games." Olympic.org. 2014. http://www.olympic.org/ancient-olympic-games.

Anderson, P. "Global Use of Alcohol, Drugs and Tobacco." *Drug and Alcohol Review* 25, no. 6 (2006): 489–502.

Barr, Andrew. *Drink: A Social History of America.* New York: Carroll & Graf, 1999.

Blanding, Michael. "There's Something about Molly: How a Supposedly Safe Party Drug Turned Lethal." *Boston Globe Magazine.* January 26, 2014. http://www.bostonglobe.com/magazine/2014/01/26/what-drug-molly-and-how-turned-lethal/1x7T7p7lGlhxCaSUj3sUwI/story.html.

"A Brief History of Methamphetamine: Methamphetamine Prevention in Vermont." Vermont Department of Health. 2014. http://healthvermont.gov/adap/meth/brief_history.aspx.

Dietler, M. "Alcohol: Anthropological/Archaeological Perspectives." *Annual Review of Anthropology* 35, no. 1 (2006): 229–49.

Dziemianowicz, Joe. "The Top 10 Pop Culture Trends of the '80s." *New York Daily News.* April 14, 2013. http://www.nydailynews.com/entertainment/joe-dziemianowicz-top

-10-80s-pop-culture-trends-article-1.1312866#ixzz33QK
RF670.

"Ecstasy Brief Outline." Narconon International. http://www
.narconon.org/drug-information/ecstasy-brief-outline.html.

"Entertainment in the Middle Ages." Lordsandladies.org. June
2014. http://www.lordsandladies.org/entertainment
-middle-ages.htm.

Fife, Steven. "Athletics, Leisure, and Entertainment in Ancient
Rome." *Ancient History Encyclopedia*. January 18, 2012. http://
www.ancient.eu.com/article/98/.

Gonzalez, David. "Will Gentrification Spoil the Birthplace
of Hip-Hop?" *New York Times*. May 21, 2007. http://www
.nytimes.com/2007/05/21/nyregion/21citywide.html.

Hattikudur, Mangesh. "5 Drinking Games of Yore." *Mental Floss*.
April 22, 2014. http://mentalfloss.com/article/16282
/drinking-games-yore.

Hebbar, J. V. "Health Benefits of Alcohol Consumption—
Ayurveda Viewpoint." Easy Ayurveda. August 8, 2011. http://
easyayurveda.com/2011/08/08/health-benefits-of-alcohol
-consumption-ayurveda-viewpoint.

"Heroin Chic." *Wikipedia*. August 25, 2014. http://en.wikipedia
.org/wiki/Heroin_chic.

The Holy Bible: New International Version. Colorado Springs:
Biblica, 2011.

Kareti, Kavitha. "Elizabethan England: Popular Amusements
and Entertainment." Springfield [Illinois] Public Schools.
http://www2.springfield.k12.il.us/schools/springfield/eliz
/amusements.html.

Lewis, Jone Johnson. "Carrie Nation: Hatchet-Wielding Saloon
Smasher." About Education: Women's History. 2014. http://
womenshistory.about.com/od/temperance/a/Carrie-Nation
.htm.

McGovern, Patrick E. *Uncorking the Past: The Quest for Wine, Beer, and Other Alcoholic Beverages.* Berkeley: University of California Press, 2009.

Meussdoerffer, Franz G. "Beer and Beer Culture in Germany." In *Liquid Bread: Beer and Brewing in Cross-Cultural Perspective,* edited by W. Schiefenhövel and H. Macbeth, 63–70. New York: Bergahn, 2011.

———. "A Comprehensive History of Beer Brewing." In *Handbook of Brewing: Processes, Technology, Markets,* edited by Hans Michael Esslinger, 1–42. Weinheim, Germany: Wiley-VCH, 2009.

"Mrs. Winslow's Soothing Syrup." Catalog record. Wood Library Museum. http://woodlibrarymuseum.org/museum /item/529/mrs.-winslow%27s-soothing-syrup.

"Nation: Rushing to a New High." *Time.* July 17, 1978.

Patrick, Charles H. *Alcohol, Culture, and Society.* 1952. Reprint, New York: AMS, 1970.

"Prehistoric Cave Etchings Created by Three-Year-Olds." *BBC News.* September 30, 2011. www.bbc.co.uk/news /entertainment-arts-15109188.

"Prehistoric Music." Copernicus Science Centre. http://www .kopernik.org.pl/en/exhibitions/archiwum-wystaw /wszystko-gra/muzyka-prehistoryczna.

"Puritan Life." *U.S. History Online Textbook.* December 1, 2014. http://www.ushistory.org/us/3d.asp.

Rabin, Dana. "Drunkenness and Responsibility for Crime in the Eighteenth Century." *Social History of Alcohol and Drugs* 22, no. 1 (Fall 2007).

Raymond, Adam K. "PCP, Quaaludes, Mescaline: What Became of Yesterday's 'It' Drugs?" *The Fix.* December 30, 2011. http://www.thefix.com/content/where-are-they-now-drugs -edition7098.

Siegel, Ronald K. *Intoxication: The Universal Drive for Mind-Altering Substances.* Rochester, VT: Park Street, 2005.

Stika, H-P. "Beer in Prehistoric Europe." In *Liquid Bread: Beer and Brewing in Cross-Cultural Perspective,* edited by Hans Michael Esslinger, 55–62. New York: Berghahn Books, 2011.

Thera, Piyadassi. *Mahāsatipaṭṭhāna Sutta: The Great Discourse on Establishing Mindfulness.* Translated by Vipassana Research Institute. Seattle: Vipassana Research Publications of America, 1996.

"Timeline: The Pill." *American Experience.* PBS. 2003. http://www.pbs.org/wgbh/amex/pill/timeline/timeline2.html.

Volkow, Nora D. "America's Addiction to Opioids: Heroin and Prescription Drug Abuse." National Institute on Drug Abuse Presentation to Senate Caucus on International Narcotics Control. May 14, 2014. http://www.drugabuse.gov/about -nida/legislative-activities/testimony-to-congress/2014 /americas-addiction-to-opioids-heroin-prescription-drug -abuse.

"What Are Petroglyphs and Who Made Them?" National Park Service. http://www.nps.gov/petr/historyculture/what.htm.

"What Did Kids in Colonial Times Do for Games and Recreation?" Answers.com. http://www.answers.com/Q /What_did_kids_in_colonial_times_do_for_games_and _recreation.

Wheadon, Bret. "Shakespeare: Life in Elizabethan Times" (slideshow). Slideshare.net. September 23, 2013. http://www .slideshare.net/bretwheadon/shakespeare-life-in -shakespearean-times.

Wilford, John Noble. "Wine Cellar, Well Aged, Is Revealed in Israel." *New York Times.* November 22, 2013. http://www .nytimes.com/2013/11/23/science/in-ruins-of-palace-a-wine -with-hints-of-cinnamon-and-top-notes-of-antiquity.html.

Chapter 2: The Craving Brain

"The Craving Brain: The Neuroscience of Uncontrollable Urges."
World Science Festival. New York. May 31, 2014. http://www
.worldsciencefestival.com/program/the_craving_brain.

Johnson, Lorie. "Adderall Addiction: Lessons from a Son's
Suicide." *CBN News*. October 23, 2013. http://www.cbn.com
/cbnnews/healthscience/2013/october/adderall-addiction
-lessons-from-a-sons-suicide.

Sibilla, Nick. "Naloxone Reverses Drug Overdoses, Saves 10,000
Lives." *Hit & Run* (blog). February 21, 2012. http://reason
.com/blog/2012/02/21/naloxone-reverses-drug-overdoses
-saves10.

Specter, Michael. "Partial Recall." *New Yorker*. May 19, 2014.
http://www.newyorker.com/magazine/2014/05/19/partial
-recall.

Chapter 3: Birds Do It, Bees Do It

"American Robin." *All About Birds*. Cornell Lab of Ornithology.
http://www.allaboutbirds.org/guide/american_robin/id.

"Basic Hedgehog Facts." Hedgehog Central. http://www
.hedgehogcentral.com/stats.shtml.

Celli, Giorgio. *Vita segreta degli animali*. Casale Monferrato, Italy:
Piemme, 1999.

Darwin, Charles. *On the Origin of Species by Means of Natural
Selection, or the Preservation of Favoured Races in the Struggle for
Life*. London: John Murray, 1859.

Derbyshire, David. "Elephants Never Forget Old Friends and Are
Social Network Experts." *Daily Mail* (London). July 27, 2011.
http://www.dailymail.co.uk/sciencetech/article-2019178
/Elephants-forget-old-friends-social-network-experts.html.

Freye, Enno. *Pharmacology and Abuse of Cocaine, Amphetamines,
Ecstasy, and Related Designer Drugs: A Comprehensive Review
on Their Mode of Action, Treatment of Abuse and Intoxication*.
Dordrecht: Springer, 2009.

Fries, Wendy C. "Keeping an Indoor Cat Happy." WebMD. http://pets.webmd.com/features/keeping-indoor-cat-happy.

Grant, V., and K. A. Grant. "Behavior of Hawkmoths on Flowers of Datura Meteloides." *Botanical Gazette* 144 (1983): 280–84.

"How Do Gorillas Play?" Berggorilla & Regenwald Direkthilfe. 2011. http://www.berggorilla.org/en/gorillas/general/social-life/how-do-gorillas-play/.

Kivi, Rose. "How Do Dolphins Play?" eHow. 2012. http://www.ehow.com/how-does_4566670_dolphins-play.html#ixzz31M1QmpfK.

"Meet the Animals: Sheep and Goats." Farm Sanctuary. http://www.farmsanctuary.org/learn/someone-not-something/sheep-goats/#.

O'Brien, Jodie Munro. "It's a Dog of a Way to Get High but Queensland Pooches Are Lapping Up Hallucinogenic Sweat from Cane Toads." *Courier-Mail* (Brisbane). December 13, 2013. http://www.couriermail.com.au/news/queensland/its-a-dog-of-a-way-to-get-high-but-queensland-pooches-are-lapping-up-hallucinogenic-sweat-from-cane-toads/story-fnihsrf2-1226783570516.

Ogilvie, Felicity. "Happy Hops Damage Poppy Crops." June 24, 2009. Australian Broadcasting Company. http://www.abc.net.au/news/2009-06-25/happy-hops-damage-poppy-crops/1332044.

"Play Behavior in Horses." My Horse University. http://www.myhorseuniversity.com/EE/December2012/Play.

"Reindeer Behavior." Reindeers.info. June 6, 2006. http://reindeers.info/reindeer_articles/reindeer-behavior/.

Rushton, Cate. "Emotional Characteristics of the Elephant." PawNation. http://animals.pawnation.com/emotional-characteristics-elephant-10845.html.

Samorini, Giorgio. *Animals and Psychedelics: The Natural World and the Instinct to Alter Consciousness.* Translated by Tami Calliope. Rochester, VT: Park Street, 2002.

Schoenian, Susan. "Sheep Behavior." Sheep 201: A Beginner's Guide to Raising Sheep. June 18, 2011. http://www.sheep101 .info/201/behavior.html.

Siegel, Ronald K. *Intoxication: The Universal Drive for Mind-Altering Substances.* Rochester, VT: Park Street, 2005.

Sweat, Rebecca. "Games You Can Play with Your Pet Bird." Birdchannel.com. 2009. http://www.birdchannel.com/bird-diet-and-health/bird -care/games-birds-play.aspx.

Veissier, I., et al. "Animals' Emotions: Studies in Sheep Using Appraisal Theories." *Animal Welfare* 18 (2009): 347–54.

"Vervet Monkey." Out to Africa with Ellen and Paul. http:// www.outtoafrica.nl/animals/engvervetmonkey.html.

Wall, Tim. "Animals Caught Doping Show No Remorse: Photos." *Discovery News.* January 18, 2013. http://news .discovery.com/animals/animals-on-drugs-pictures-130118 .html.

"Wallaby." *National Geographic.* http://animals.national geographic.com/animals/mammals/wallaby.

Wolford, Ben. "Do Dolphins Get High? BBC Cameras Catch Dolphins Chewing on Pufferfish Toxins." *International Science Times.* December 30, 2013. http://www.isciencetimes .com/articles/6595/20131230/dolphins-high-bbc-cameras -catch-chewing-pufferfish.htm.

Chapter 4: The High Life

Brown, Brené. *The Gifts of Imperfection: Let Go of Who You Think You're Supposed to Be and Embrace Who You Are.* Center City, MN: Hazelden, 2010.

Glatz, Carol. "In Latest Interview, Pope Francis Reveals Top 10 Secrets to Happiness." Catholic News Service. July 29, 2014. http://www.catholicnews.com/data/stories/cns/1403144 .htm.

"History of Happiness: Socrates." Pursuit of Happiness. http://www.pursuit-of-happiness.org/history-of-happiness/socrates.

"How to Achieve Happiness and the Unsung Heroes of Compassion." The Website of His Holiness the 14th Dalai Lama of Tibet. February 24, 2014. http://www.dalailama.com/news/post/1083-how-to-achieve-happiness-and-the-unsung-heroes-of-compassion.

Rubin, Gretchen. *The Happiness Project: Or Why I Spent a Year Trying to Sing in the Morning, Clean My Closets, Fight Right, Read Aristotle, and Generally Have More Fun.* New York: Harper, 2009.

Tolle, Eckhart. *Stillness Speaks.* New York: New World Library, 2003.

Pleasure Principle #1: Move

Bertheussen, G. F., et al. "Associations between Physical Activity and Physical and Mental Health: A HUNT 3 Study." *Medicine and Science in Sports and Exercise* 43, no. 7 (July 2011): 1220–28. http://www.ncbi.nlm.nih.gov/pubmed/21131869.

Brody, Jane. "To Keep Moving, Look Beyond the Physical." *New York Times.* March 8, 2010. http://www.nytimes.com/2010/03/09/health/09brod.html.

Reynolds, Gretchen. "How Exercise Helps Us Tolerate Pain." *Well* (blog). *New York Times.* August 13, 2014. http://well.blogs.nytimes.com/2014/08/13/how-exercise-helps-us-tolerate-pain/.

Sibold, Jeremy S., and Kathleen M. Berg. "Mood Enhancement Persists for Up to 12 Hours Following Aerobic Exercise: A Pilot Study." *Perceptual and Motor Skills* 111, no. 2 (October 2010): 333–42. http://www.amsciepub.com/doi/abs/10.2466/02.06.13.15.PMS.111.5.333-342.

"Stress Management: Approaches for Preventing and Reducing Stress." Harvard Health Publications. http://www.harvardhealthcontent.com/HealthyLifestyle/70,SC0211?Page=Section1.

Pleasure Principle #2: Restore

Brody, S. "Blood Pressure Reactivity to Stress Is Better for People Who Recently Had Penile-Vaginal Intercourse Than for People Who Had Other or No Sexual Activity." *Biological Psychology* (February 2006).

Burleson, M. H., W. R. Trevathan, and M. Todd. "In the Mood for Love or Vice Versa? Exploring the Relations among Sexual Activity, Physical Affection, Affect, and Stress in the Daily Lives of Mid-Aged Women." *Archives of Sexual Behavior* (June 2007).

Coelho, Paulo. *Manuscript Found in Accra: A Novel.* Translated by Margaret Jull Costa. New York: Knopf, 2013.

Denes, Amanda, and Tamara D. Afifi. "Pillow Talk and Cognitive Decision-Making Processes: Exploring the Influence of Orgasm and Alcohol on Communication after Sexual Activity." *Communication Monographs* 81, no. 3 (June 2014): 333–58. http://www.tandfonline.com/doi/abs/10.1080/03637751.2014.926377#.

Ditzen, B., et al. "Effects of Different Kinds of Couple Interaction on Cortisol and Heart Rate Responses to Stress in Women." *Psychoneuroendocrinology* (June 2007).

Khalsa, Sat Bir Singh, and Jodie Gould. *Your Brain on Yoga.* A Harvard Medical School Guide. New York: Rosetta, 2012.

Leder, Steven Z. *More Money Than God: Living a Rich Life without Losing Your Soul.* Chicago: Bonus Books, 2003.

Ramaswamy, Sandhiya. "The Benefits of Ayurveda Self-Massage, 'Abhyanga.'" Chopra Centered Lifestyle. http://www.chopra.com/ccl/the-benefits-of-ayurveda-self-massage-abhyanga.

Treadway, Michael T., and S. W. Lazar. "Meditation and Neuroplasticity: Using Mindfulness to Change the Brain." *Assessing Mindfulness and Acceptance Processes in Clients: Illuminating the Theory and Practice of Change*, edited by Ruth A. Baer, 186–205. Oakland: Context, 2010.

Pleasure Principle #3: Connect

Eger, Isaac. "'I Got Net': Exploring New York Through Pickup Basketball." *New York Times*. July 11, 2012. http://www .nytimes.com/2012/07/12/sports/basketball/a-new-arrival -explores-new-york-through-pickup-basketball.html.

Gladwell, Malcolm. *Outliers: The Story of Success*. New York: Little Brown, 2007.

Pleasure Principle #4: Create

Sacks, Oliver. *Musicophilia: Tales of Music and the Brain*. New York: Knopf, 2007.

Verghese, Joe, et al. "Leisure Activities and the Risk of Dementia in the Elderly." *New England Journal of Medicine* 348, no. 25 (2003): 2508–16.

Pleasure Principle #5: Celebrate

Berk, Lee, et al. "Humor Similar to Meditation Enhances EEG Power Spectral Density of Gamma Wave Band Activity (31-40Hz) and Synchrony (684.5)." *FASEB Journal* 28, no. 1, supplement (2014): 684–85.

"By the Numbers: The American Vacation." *CBS Sunday Morning*. August 3, 2014. http://www.cbsnews.com/news/by-the -numbers-the-american-vacation.

"Expedia 2013 Vacation Deprivation Survey." Expedia. November 2013. http://viewfinder.expedia.com/docs /default-source/downloadable-pr-docs/stor-16189_vacation _deprivation.pdf?sfvrsn=2.

Melton, Glennon Doyle. "Give Me Gratitude or Give Me Debt."
Momastery (blog). August 11, 2014. http://momastery.com
/blog/2014/08/11/give-liberty-give-debt.

Preidt, Robert. "Laughter May Work Like Meditation in the
Brain: Study Monitored Brain Waves of People Watching
Different Types of Videos." *HealthDay*. April 27, 2014. http://
www.webmd.com/mental-health/news/20140427/laughter
-may-work-like-meditation-in-the-brain.

Strauss-Blasche, G., C. Ekmekcioglu, and W. Marktl. "Does
Vacation Enable Recuperation? Changes in Well-Being
Associated with Time Away from Work." *Occupational
Medicine* (April 2000). http://www.ncbi.nlm.nih.gov/pubmed
/10912359.

"U.S. Only Advanced Economy That Does Not Guarantee
Paid Vacation or Holidays: Report Shows That 1 in 4 U.S.
Workers Have No Paid Vacation." Center for Economic and
Policy Research. May 2007. http://www.cepr.net/documents
/publications/nvn-summary.pdf.

Pleasure Principle #6: Give

"The Humane Society of the United States." Great Nonprofits.
http://greatnonprofits.org/org/the-humane-society-of-the
-united-states.

"ICAN, International Cancer Advocacy Network." Great
Nonprofits. http://greatnonprofits.org/org/ican
-international-cancer-advocacy-network.

Kristof, Nicholas D., and Sheryl WuDunn. *A Path Appears:
Transforming Lives, Creating Opportunity*. New York: Knopf,
2014.

Also of Interest

Choosing a Good Life: Lessons from People
Who Have Found Their Place in the World
Ali Berman
Ever wonder why some people seem to be at peace despite the ups and
downs daily life can bring, while others are restless even in seemingly
ideal circumstances? In *Choosing a Good Life*, Ali Berman explores what
it means to be at peace with ourselves, our choices, and the world
around us in all its glorious chaos. Order no. 7538 (softcover). Also
available as an e-book.

The Next Happy: Let Go of the Life You Planned
and Find a New Way Forward
Tracey Cleantis
The reality is that no matter how positive our outlook or how tena-
cious our approach, our dreams simply do not always come true. When
the best option is to let go of the life you planned for yourself and
find a new path, a world of possibilities can surprisingly open up. This
book provides the guidance and support to help you discover the next
happy. Order no. 7768. Also available as an e-book.

The Gifts of Imperfection: Let Go of Who You Think
You're Supposed to Be and Embrace Who You Are
Brené Brown, Ph.D., L.M.S.W.
This *New York Times* best-seller by Brené Brown, Ph.D., a leading expert
on shame, blends original research with honest storytelling and helps
readers move from "What will people think?" to "I am enough." Order
no. 2545. Also available as an e-book.

For more information or to order these or other resources from
Hazelden Publishing, call **800-328-9000** or visit **hazelden.org/bookstore**.